DIAGNOSTIC REPORTS

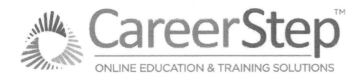

ONLINE EDUCATION & TRAINING SOLUTIONS

Career Step, LLC
Phone: 801.489.9393
Toll-Free: 800.246.7837
Fax: 801.491.6645
careerstep.com

This text companion contains a snapshot of the online program content converted to a printed format. Please note that the online training program is constantly changing and improving and is always the source of the most up-to-date information.

Product Number: HG-PR-11-008
Generation Date: March 13, 2015

TABLE OF CONTENTS

UNIT 1

Introduction

INTRODUCTION TO DIAGNOSTIC REPORTS

Learning Objectives

Diagnostic Report Basics – Students will be able to identify the basic elements of a diagnostic report, including identification of an illness/condition and any present therapeutic components.

Diagnostic Specialties – Students will be able to use common terms and references related to the specialties of emergency room, physical medicine, radiology, and pathology.

Diagnostic reports are, as the name implies, reports where identification of an illness or other problem is made by examination of the symptoms. This, of course, is a very general definition. In this module you will be exposed to a variety of specialties or subspecialties that can loosely be clumped together in a category of reports that are diagnostic in nature. The specialties in this diagnostic grouping also have a therapeutic component. For example, let's say a patient comes into the ER for difficulty breathing. A diagnosis is made of reactive airway disease, a breathing treatment is administered, recommendation is made for followup with a pulmonologist. This patient was both diagnosed and treated by the ER. Radiology is frequently broken down into diagnostic and therapeutic types of radiology. For example, bone x-rays are typically diagnostic, while a gamma knife surgery is radiation therapy. Likewise, physical medicine and pathology have both diagnostic and therapeutic application. For our purposes we are earmarking them all "diagnostic reports."

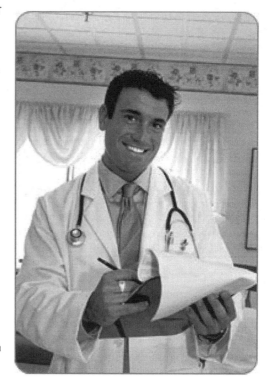

The subspecialties covered in this module include:

- Emergency Room
- Physical Medicine
- Radiology
- Pathology

Each unit begins with an explanation of the specific subspecialty, a targeted language workshop and review, a variety of sample reports, a report with an accompanying audio, and a unit test to finish it up. Upon completion of this module, you should have a firm understanding of diagnostic reports, not to mention an expanded word list and additional reference materials for use in the practicum portions of this training program.

UNIT 2

Emergency Room

EMERGENCY ROOM – INTRODUCTION

The term *emergency room* might be a tad outdated and will likely be replaced with *emergency department*, but the meaning is clear (and the terms *emergency room* and *emergency department* will be used interchangeably throughout this unit).

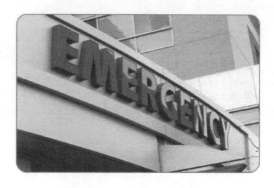

The emergency department sees a variety of afflictions on any given day. Some common ailments or conditions treated in an ER include (but are not limited to):

- fractures
- motor vehicle accidents
- heart attacks, chest pain
- burns
- poisoning/hazardous materials exposure
- gastritis
- ear infection
- laceration
- unconsciousness
- allergic reactions

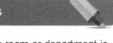

Highlights

An emergency room or department is an area in a hospital or clinic that is staffed and equipped to provide emergency care to persons requiring immediate medical treatment.

Upon arrival at an emergency department, people typically are evaluated in triage, a medical screening of the nature and severity of illness to determine relative priority for treatment. Individuals with serious illnesses are then admitted to the department more rapidly than those with less severe symptoms or injuries. After initial assessment and treatment in the emergency room, patients are admitted to the hospital, transferred to a specialty hospital, or discharged.

EMERGENCY ROOM OVERVIEW

Emergency rooms are open 24 hours a day, 7 days a week. Through hospital emergency rooms, patients have access to healthcare outside of routine clinic or physician hours. Emergency rooms also are the gateway for immediate access to diagnostic tests, equipment and interventions (such as laboratories, operating suites, CT and MRI), and, through physician hospital affiliations, a wide variety of medical specialists.

True "emergency" room visits generally fall into two categories.

- Acute exacerbations of underlying problems
- Trauma

In reality, the emergency room also treats numerous patients for non-emergencies such as sore throats and ear infections. Non-emergency treatment in the emergency room occurs because many patients do not have a primary physician, medical insurance, or (in some cases) common sense to seek treatment in a more routine care setting.

Ultimately, the mission of emergency room medicine is to provide "triage" care and not to be a final solution for medical care. **Triage care** is making an assessment of the patient's immediate need, stabilizing the "emergency," and then (when necessary) referring the patient to an appropriate setting for ongoing and/or followup care.

NON-EMERGENCY EMERGENCY ROOM CARE

For 10–15 hours a day, emergency rooms are the only game in town. Although many cities have added emergency clinics or urgent care centers, for many people the only choice for obtaining medical care outside of regular business hours is through the emergency room.

EMERGENCY ROOM LANGUAGE WORKSHOP

Dictators frequently use slang, jargon, or shortened forms, and we hardly even recognize them as such because they have become so commonplace. Nowhere is this truer than in the emergency room. While abbreviated forms are often acceptable, the same thing is not necessarily true of slang. That said, in some types of medical reports, such as ER notes, clinic notes, and nurses' notes, many slang and jargon terms are acceptable. Simple shortened forms are even more widely acceptable.

Whether or not slang or abbreviated words are expanded in ER reports will be determined most likely by the client through account instructions. Because ER has a language of its own, it is important to be familiar with the jargon associated with the emergency room visit. The following is a list, albeit not exhaustive, of some common emergency medicine and general medical slang terms and definitions. We are also including a list of common ER abbreviations. Please note that many of these abbreviations have multiple acceptable expansions. The ones listed below are the most common ER-related expansions. The *Stedman's Abbreviations, Acronyms & Symbols, third edition* and the *Stedman's Emergency Medicine Words* books were used as references for this lesson. These resource books are highly recommended.

Common ER Slang Terms

Slang	Expansion
alk phos/alk P-tase	alkaline phosphatase
ambo	transporting ambulance
Ambu	ambu bag, manual resuscitative device
appy	appendectomy
bagging	artificial respiration performed with a respirator bag, such as an ambu bag
bag/banana bag	bag of IV fluids given to alcoholics or patients with nutritional deficiencies or chemical imbalances; named because of its yellow color, it contains multivitamins, folate, thiamine, and sugar
bicarb	bicarbonate
bili	bilirubin
Binky test	ability of an infant to evidence basic stability and an interest in "the important things in life" by placidly sucking on a binky
bleed	hemorrhage
champagne tap	clear tap; no blood
chem dep	chemical dependency
crit	hematocrit
eos	eosinophils
epi	epinephrine
epi sick	pale, green, nauseous, chest-pounding, tachycardic appearance of patient who has received aggressive subcutaneous epinephrine therapy for anaphylaxis or status asthmaticus
epis	epithelial cells
four H's	hypoxemia, hypoglycemia, hypovolemia, and high bladder
gorked	obtunded or not alert, either acutely or chronically
HOD	heroin overdose
hypo	hypodermic injection
lac	laceration
lap coly	laparoscopic cholecystectomy
leuks	leukocytes
lido	lidocaine
lytes	electrolytes

mag	magnesium
monos	monocytes
neuts	neutrophils
nitro paste	Nitrol, nitroglycerin paste
perfed appy	ruptured appendix
quant beta/Q-beta	quantitative beta HCG
rule of 9's	for assessing percentage of body surface burned
satting/sat	oxygen saturation
sed rate	sedimentation rate
serum/urine ozm(s)	serum/urine osmolality/osmolalities (lab)
stepdown unit	a monitored setting, not as intense as any type of ICU
sux/sucks	succinylcholine
Tee-3/TN-3/Ty-3	Tylenol No. 3
tox	toxicology
traked	endotracheally intubated
triple A	abdominal aortic aneurysm, AAA
tweak score	scale for assessing alcoholism dependence
vitamin H	ER short form for Haldol

Common ER Abbreviations

Abbreviation	Expansion
AAA	abdominal aortic aneurysm
ABCs	airway, breathing, circulation
ABG	arterial blood gas
ABW	adjusted body weight
ACLS	advanced cardiac life support
AEIOU TIPS	a mnemonic for altered mental status check
ALS	advanced life support
AMA	against medical advice
amp	ampule
AO X3	alert and oriented X 3
ATLS	advanced trauma life support
BF	black female
BLS	basic life support
BM	black male/bowel movement
BMI	body mass index
BSA	body surface area
BVM	bag-valve-mask
CAPD	continuous ambulatory peritoneal dialysis

CCU	coronary care unit
CID	cervical immobilization device
CPR	cardiopulmonary resuscitation
CVA	cerebrovascular accident
D5 or D5W	5% dextrose in water
DNI	do not intubate
DNR	do not resuscitate
DOA	dead on arrival
ECC	emergency cardiac care
EMS	emergency medical service
EMT	emergency medical technician
ESR	erythrocyte sedimentation rate
ETA	estimated time of arrival
FACEP	Fellow of the American College of Emergency Physicians
FDIU	fetal death in utero
FHT	fetal heart tone
FOOSH	fall onto outstretched hand
GCS	Glasgow Coma Scale
GSW	gunshot wound
HF	Hispanic female
HM	Hispanic male
IABP	intraaortic balloon pump
IBW	ideal body weight
IM	intramuscular
IO	intraosseous
IV	intravenous
IVDA	intravenous drug abuser
IVP	intravenous push
JONES	a mnemonic for assessment of rheumatic fever
LMA	laryngeal mask airway
LOC	loss of consciousness
LR	lactated Ringer
LWBS	left without being seen
M&M	morbidity and mortality
MVA	motor vehicle accident
NG	nasogastric (tube)
NS	normal saline
NSR	normal sinus rhythm
OD	overdose

OPQRST	a mnemonic for pain evaluation
PALS	pediatric advanced life support
PQRST	a mnemonic to quickly evaluate chest pain
RRR	regular rate and rhythm
TTP	trauma transport protocol
WD	withdrawal
WF	white female
WM	white male
WNL	within normal limits
WNR	within normal range
WO	weeks old
WOB	work of breathing
WX	wound of exit
XKO	not knocked out
XRT	radiation therapy
Y/N	yes/no
YO	years old

Career Step is not affiliated with Lippincott Williams & Wilkins. *Stedman's Medical Dictionary* is just one of many good sources available and is used here for illustrative purposes.

REVIEW: EMERGENCY ROOM LANGUAGE

MULTIPLE CHOICE.
Choose the best answer.

1. The slang term appy means (⊘ appendectomy, ⊘ application).

2. The slang term for bicarbonate is (⊘ binate, ⊘ bicarb).

3. Routinely the term (⊘ bleed, ⊘ rrhage) is used for hemorrhage.

4. A triple A or AAA is an (⊘ abdominal, ⊘ anterior) aortic aneurysm.

5. The slang term sed rate means (⊘ spoken, ⊘ sedimentation) rate.

FILL IN THE BLANK.
Using the word(s) in the box, enter the appropriate term in the space provided.

1. BLS – _____ life support

2. ETA – estimated time of _____

3. LOC – loss of _____

4. CPR – cardiopulmonary _____

5. LR – _____ Ringer

6. IVP – _____ push

7. RRR – regular rate and _____

8. XRT – radiation _____

9. M&M – morbidity and _____

10. WNR – within normal _____

arrival
basic
consciousness
intravenous
lactated
mortality
range
resuscitation
rhythm
therapy

TRUE/FALSE.
Mark the following true or false.

1. NSR stands for normal sinus rate.

    ⊘ true

    ⊘ false

2. IO stands for intraorally.

    ⊘ true

    ⊘ false

3. DNI stands for do not intubate.

    ⊘ true

    ⊘ false

4. GCS is the abbreviation for a gun shot that is critical.

    ⊘ true

    ⊘ false

5. CVA stands for a cerebrovascular accident.

    ⊘ true

    ⊘ false

EMERGENCY ROOM REPORTS

Emergency room reports are the descriptive reports of emergency room visits. They include a brief history, physical examination pertinent to the problem, any tests performed and treatment given, and finally the disposition and/or followup instructions. Because emergency rooms focus on identifying and stabilizing the "emergency" problem and not treating the whole health of the patient, emergency room reports usually focus on documenting only what is pertinent to the current visit. Note that the patient's medical history may be pertinent in many cases since the ER doctor often needs to understand a patient's history to understand their current problem.

With ER reports the specialty is ER and the work type is ER. These are not generally classified as discharge summary or history and physical reports, but simply ER or Emergency Room reports.

As you can imagine, emergency room report transcription editing is diverse and interesting. It can involve documenting care for anything—a broken finger, a heart attack, a peanut in the nose, an acute asthma attack, or a psychotic episode. ER reports tend to be relatively short (about one page) as the function of an emergency room is "triage" and not to provide in-depth specialized treatment. Emergency room terminology covers the terminology basics across many specialties but does not require exhaustive, in-depth familiarity with medical specialties. For this reason, the terminology is relatively easy to learn.

EMERGENCY ROOM REPORT 1

HISTORY: This 44-year-old female complains of abdominal pain since yesterday. It is crampy, and it is worse with drinking liquid or eating foods. She has no prior history of similar pain. She has had vomiting 3 to 4 times today and 3 to 4 watery bowel movements today. She is uncertain whether or not she has had fevers. She has had no recent travel, no ill contacts, no spoiled foods, no dysuria or increased urinary frequency. Last menstrual period was December 11 and was normal. She is gravida 3, para 3.

PAST MEDICAL HISTORY: Negative.

PAST SURGICAL HISTORY: Appendectomy.

MEDICATIONS: None.

SOCIAL HISTORY: The patient is a smoker.

ALLERGIES: None known.

PHYSICAL EXAMINATION: Vital signs: Temperature 97.5, pulse 80, respirations 16, blood pressure 128/80. This is an uncomfortable Caucasian female who is having retching and dry heaves on initial evaluation by myself. Head, eyes, ears, nose, and throat exam is unremarkable. Lungs have mild expiratory rhonchi bilaterally. However, the patient is in no respiratory distress. The heart has a regular rate and rhythm without murmurs. The abdomen is mildly tender in the left upper quadrant. The abdomen is, however, quite soft, with active bowel sounds. There is no CVA tenderness. There is no rebound or guarding. Rectal examination is heme negative[1]. Extremities are unremarkable.

Reexamination at 8:10 p.m., after several liters of fluid and some IV Inapsine[2] reveals no abdominal tenderness whatsoever. The patient's nausea is resolved.

DIAGNOSTIC DATA: White blood cell count 7.8, hematocrit 35.5, sodium 134, potassium 4.1, chloride 105, bicarb 24, glucose 97, BUN 11, creatinine 0.7.[3] Urinalysis is negative. Amylase 63. A 4-way of the abdomen is unremarkable. An echo[4] shows normal sinus rhythm and no acute ischemic changes.

FINAL DIAGNOSIS: Vomiting and abdominal pain.

Footnotes:

1. 1.As you know from your studies of root words in the Medical Word Building module, the root hem/a, hem/o, hemat/o means blood. Rectal exam is heme negative meaning no blood was detected on rectal exam.
2. 2.Inapsine is a trademark preparation of droperidol, an antiemetic (among other things).
3. 3.Oftentimes the lab values are hard to hear or difficult to decipher with complete certainty. It is a good idea to check lab values to make sure they are plausible—one way to do this is to reference a normal lab values document or website. Simply do a web search for "normal lab values" for your pick of references.
4. 4.Slang for echocardiogram. Some accounts require this be expanded, but many have you edit as dictated—the meaning is completely clear.

SPELLING.
Determine if the following words are spelled correctly. If the spelling is correct, leave the word as it has already been entered. If the spelling is incorrect, provide the correct spelling.

1. caucasion _____

2. appindectomy _____

3. creatinine _____

4. murmer _____

5. heme _____

MULTIPLE CHOICE.

Choose the best answer.

1. Lungs have mild (○ inspiratory, ○ expiratory) rhonchi bilaterally.

2. Inapsine was given to the patient (○ orally, ○ intravenously).

3. The patient (○ has, ○ has not) had recent painful or difficult urination.

4. The patient is gravida (○ 3, ○ 6).

5. On exam, the patient was (○ febrile, ○ afebrile).

EMERGENCY ROOM REPORT 2

CHIEF COMPLAINT: Fall.

HISTORY OF PRESENT ILLNESS: The patient is a 60-year-old male with a history of having been up on a ladder painting. The ladder started to fall, and he rode the ladder down to the ground, upon which he fell forward, striking his face on the rungs of the ladder. He was not knocked out but comes in complaining of pain primarily over his nose, upper lip, and his teeth.

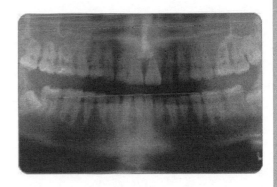

Panelipse is a facial/dental x-ray that shows an overview of all teeth and their surrounding areas.

PHYSICAL EXAMINATION: A 60-year-old male in no acute distress, awake, alert, and oriented. Neck is supple and nontender. Back is nontender. Pelvis is stable. No crepitus is palpable. Extremities all move full range of motion without deficit.[1] Facially, the patient shows a 3-cm laceration to the right side of his nose, a 1.5-cm laceration midline of his upper lip, and a 1-cm laceration to the right cheek. Other smaller abrasions are noted as well.

X-rays of the nasal and facial bones show no signs of fracture. Panelipse shows no fracture of the mandible or maxilla.

DIAGNOSIS.

1. Multiple facial lacerations, contusions.
2. Dental avulsions.

ED TREATMENT: The patient's facial lacerations were anesthetized with 1% Xylocaine, prepped with Betadine, and subsequently closed with a total of eleven 6-0[2] Prolene sutures. The patient was given a wound care sheet and advised to have sutures removed in 5 days. Dr. Smith[3] came in to evaluate the patient for his dental injuries and arranged a subsequent dental followup.

Footnotes:

1. [1] This sentence doesn't read well, but meaning is clear and it should be edited as dictated, unless account allows minor editing.
2. [2] It would be confusing and hard to read if numerals were used exclusively in this statement: 11 6-0 Prolene sutures. Therefore, one of the numbers has been spelled out.
3. [3] In this report, and all reports in this module, information has been changed to protect patient identity.

MULTIPLE CHOICE
Choose the best answer.

1. The lower jawbone.
   - ○ maxila
   - ○ maxilla
   - ○ mandable
   - ○ mandible

2. The upper jawbone.
   - ○ maxilla
   - ○ maxilia
   - ○ mandable
   - ○ mandible

3. Noise or vibration produced by rubbing bone or degenerated cartilage surfaces together.
   - ○ crepitis
   - ○ crepitous
   - ○ crepitus
   - ○ crepitas

4. Adjusted or located in relation to surroundings or circumstances.
   - ○ oriented
   - ○ awake
   - ○ alert
   - ○ distress

5. A lack or deficiency.
   - ○ defecet
   - ○ defecit
   - ○ deficet
   - ○ deficit

True/False.
Mark the following true or false.

1. The patient was knocked out upon striking the ground.

   ○ true

   ○ false

2. The patient's laceration on his right cheek was 3 cm long.

   ○ true

   ○ false

3. There were no signs of facial fracture.

   ○ true

   ○ false

4. The patient had dental injuries.

   ○ true

   ○ false

5. A total of 6 sutures were used to close the facial lacerations.

   ○ true

   ○ false

EMERGENCY ROOM REPORT 3

This is an 89-year-old male who has a history of COPD and GERD who states he has been having some worsening problems with his breathing since stopping his prednisone taper and Levaquin, which he finished today. He also reports having some increasing belching and stomach acid over the same time period.

MEDICATIONS: The patient does take Azmacort, Serevent, Aciphex, and guaifenesin.

PHYSICAL EXAMINATION[1]
VITAL SIGNS: Please see the nurse's note.
HEART: Regular rate and rhythm without murmur.
LUNGS: Moderately decreased breath sounds noted.
ABDOMEN: Positive bowel sounds, tender in the epigastric area. No rebound, no guarding, no masses.
EXTREMITIES: No pedal edema noted.

ED COURSE: The patient was instructed to use his Combivent inhaler and felt significantly better. We did do a cardiac workup on him.

EKG was performed, which showed a sinus rhythm with a rate of 69. He does have a first-degree AV block as well as some left ventricular hypertrophy, all seen on prior EKGs.

AP and lateral chest x-ray was performed, which showed no acute changes from chest x-ray done June 7, 2002.

A complete CBC with automated differential WBC count shows a white blood cell count of 7700[2] without a left shift. Hemoglobin and hematocrit are stable at 12.2 and 36.1. Comprehensive metabolic profile was within normal limits.

We also did cardiac enzymes, which included a total CPK of 134 and quantitative troponin of 0.02.

DIAGNOSES:

1. Gastroesophageal reflux disease. We will bump up his Aciphex to 20 mg twice daily.
2. Chronic obstructive pulmonary disease. Patient instructed to use Combivent inhaler as his main inhaler and albuterol only on an as needed basis, q.6 h.[3]
3. First-degree AV block and left ventricular hypertrophy. He will follow up with his cardiologist as scheduled.

Patient will be seen as needed in the ER.

Footnotes:

1. 1.Physical exams, as you know from the "Healthcare Documentation" module, can be formatted a number of ways. Quite frequently in ER reports the subheadings are left justified, single spaced, and ALL CAPPED.
2. 2.This is also acceptably edited as 7,700. When there are 5 numerals in a value, it is preferred to always use a comma (83,000 and not 83000), unless a decimal is used, then no comma (87654.32 and not 87,654.32). These, of course, are general style preferences.
3. 3.The designation q.6 h. translates to every 6 hours. There is typically no space between the q. and the numeric value, but one between the number and the unit of measurement (hours or days, etc.—q.4 days instead of q. 4 days or q. 4d.)

SPELLING.
Determine if the following words are spelled correctly. If the spelling is correct, leave the word as it has already been entered. If the spelling is incorrect, provide the correct spelling.

1. cardiac _____

2. hemaglobin _____

3. Acifex _____

4. epicastric _____

5. hypratrophy _____

True/False.
Mark the following true or false.

1. The patient had a heart rate of 69.

    ○ true

    ○ false

2. No heart murmur was heard.

    ○ true

    ○ false

3. The patient had a second-degree AV block.

    ○ true

    ○ false

4. AP and lateral chest x-ray was performed, which showed acute changes from chest x-ray done June 7, 2002.

    ○ true

    ○ false

5. The patient had right ventricular hypertrophy.

    ○ true

    ○ false

SUBJECTIVE: Patient is a 22-year-old white male with no significant past medical history who presents to the emergency room tonight with a head injury. He was attending a professional bull-riding contest when he was involved in an altercation with a rodeo clown. He was hit on the left side of his head with an unknown object, possibly a guitar-shaped belt buckle. He denies any loss of consciousness.

He did drive home and noted some bleeding, so he drove himself to the ER. He admits drinking alcohol earlier tonight. He denies any drug use. He complains of slight pain at the site[1] of trauma, otherwise no headache. He has blurry vision, "secondary to alcohol," and says he always has this when he drinks. No speech problems. No weakness, or any other focal neurologic deficits or complaints.

PAST MEDICAL HISTORY: Negative.

ALLERGIES: PENICILLIN CAUSES RASH.

FAMILY HISTORY: Noncontributory.

SOCIAL HISTORY: He does smoke. He drinks 2–3 times per week. No drugs.

REVIEW OF SYSTEMS: No fevers, chills. No headaches. No chest pain, shortness of breath. No abdominal pain, nausea, or vomiting. Otherwise, he feels well.

PHYSICAL EXAM: Blood pressure is 110/66, pulse 88, respiratory rate 18, temperature was not obtained. GENERAL: He is alert and oriented, smells of alcohol. He is covered in blood. Head is notable for a left temporal artery laceration about 1 cm with blood actively spurting from it, and a very small laceration to his left cheek. NECK: Slight tenderness in the mid cervical spine. HEART: Regular rate and rhythm. LUNGS: Clear to auscultation bilaterally. ABDOMEN: Soft, nontender, nondistended. Good bowel sounds. EXTREMITIES: No edema. NEUROLOGIC: Pupils are equally round and reactive to light. Extraocular muscles are intact. Strength and sensation are intact. He is alert and oriented x3. SKIN: He does have a 1-cm laceration across the left temple with arterial bleeding. This was closed with 5-0 Vicryl interrupted sutures after pressure had limited the bleeding. Cheek laceration was closed using Steri-Strips. Both procedures were done by the surgery resident on call at the time.

LABORATORY AND X-RAY: Automated CBC: White count was 5.8, hemoglobin 14.2, platelets 238, coags were essentially normal. Alcohol level was 192.[2]

No obvious fractures are visualized on 2-view C-spine x-rays. CT of the head did show some air adjacent to the temporal bone, but otherwise no fractures or intracranial lesions or bleeds.

ASSESSMENT: Head trauma. As noted above, his temporal scalp laceration was closed by the surgeons with 5-0 Vicryl interrupted sutures. No evidence of further bleeding. C-spine film was negative. I did discuss with him that I did not see any fracture but would have the radiologist read it tomorrow, and we will call him if any abnormalities are found. He does have some air next to the temporal bone on CT scan, which is not surprising, given the trauma to this area, but there is no obvious fracture or intracranial problems. We did have somebody obtain a ride for him, given his alcohol level. The police obviously interviewed the patient in the admitting area. He was given head trauma precautions. His friend is to check on him every 2 hours, looking for vomiting, increased confusion, drowsiness, dizziness, arm or leg weakness, unequal pupils. He is to return if he has increasing headaches or above symptoms. He is to return if he has increasing redness, purulent drainage, or bleeding or pain near the laceration site. He is also to return to the admitting area in 7–8 days for suture removal.

The patient is aware of the above instructions. We did discuss it with his friend as well, and he was discharged to home in stable condition.

Footnotes:

1. 1. This was originally dictated as "sight of trauma," but the correct phrase is "site of trauma." Using "sight" would mean that he gets slight pain when he sees trauma, as opposed to the physical location or "site." These words are pronounced exactly the same; it is important to make sure you are using the correct term.
2. 2. Blood alcohol levels are often dictated like this, "one-ninety-two," and it is acceptable to edit them as done in this report (192). However, his actual BAC (blood alcohol content) is 0.192%. BAC is measured in mass per volume and 0.192% translates to 1.92 grams of alcohol per 1000 grams of blood. Currently in the U.S., the legal BAC level is 0.08%.

FILL IN THE BLANK.
Using the word(s) in the box, enter the appropriate term in the space provided.

1. The patient is to return to the ER if he has _____ drainage.
2. The patient's _____ scalp laceration was closed with Vicryl.
3. CT of the head showed no _____ lesions.
4. Patient denied loss of _____ .
5. The lungs were clear to _____ bilaterally.

auscultation
consciousness
intracranial
purulent
temporal

TRUE/FALSE.
Mark the following true or false.

1. The patient does not need to return unless he has problems with the laceration site.

    ⚪ true

    ⚪ false

2. CT scan revealed no obvious fracture.

    ⚪ true

    ⚪ false

3. The patient had a blood alcohol content level past the legal limit.

    ⚪ true

    ⚪ false

4. The head wound was closed with Steri-Strips.

    ⚪ true

    ⚪ false

5. The patient experienced blurry vision.

    ⚪ true

    ⚪ false

EMERGENCY ROOM REPORT 5

CHIEF COMPLAINT: Chest pain.

HPI: The patient is a 50-year-old female who states that today she felt an episode around 7:45 this morning where she became very shaky and developed some squeezing pressure in her chest. She felt like her heart was actually being squeezed. She stated that the tightness lasted approximately a minute and then resolved. She may have had some associated sweating with this. She denies any nausea or radiating arm, neck, jaw or back pain.

CARDIAC RISK FACTORS FOR THIS PATIENT: Prior history of myocardial infarction. Positive history for tobacco use. Positive history for family history.[1] Negative for diabetes. Negative for known hypertension. Negative for known cholesterol elevation.

PULMONARY EMBOLI RISK FACTORS: Negative for prior history of DVT or pulmonary emboli. Negative history of recent surgery, trauma or travel. Patient does not have a known history of blood abnormality or cancer. Patient does not take oral birth control medication. Positive risk factor for tobacco.

Of concern with this patient is the fact that approximately 14 years ago she had a myocardial infarction and has not been on a daily aspirin, beta blocker, or ACE inhibitor since that time. She has not had her cholesterol checked, and is not on any cholesterol-lowering medications either.

Patient states that her myocardial infarction, which she had 14 years ago, was quite different than[2] what she noted today. In particular, she had a significantly different type of chest tightness, and she was very diaphoretic during her cardiac event in the past. Patient states that the episode that she had this morning, which lasted a minute, repeated itself approximately two[3] other times, but lasted for shorter periods of time. She denies any current symptoms at the time of this examination.

OBJECTIVE FINDINGS:
VITAL SIGNS: Pulse 120, respirations 32, blood pressure 171/72.
GENERAL: Patient is alert and oriented x3. No distress.
HEART: Regular rate and rhythm. Not tachycardic on my exam.
LUNGS: Clear to auscultation bilaterally.
ABDOMEN: Positive bowel sounds, nontender, nondistended, no organomegaly. No masses. No bruits. No guarding. Mildly obese. No hepatojugular reflux noted.
NECK: No JVD. No thyromegaly noted.
EXTREMITIES: No pedal edema noted. Dorsal pedal, posterior tibial, and radial pulses strong and regular bilaterally. No palpable leg cords were noted. Negative Homans' sign.[4]

EMERGENCY DEPARTMENT WORKUP: We did do a cardiac workup on this individual, in light of her prior history and the somewhat similar history. Patient had an EKG with a sinus rhythm with a rate of 97. She did have an intraventricular conduction defect with a QRS of 122. Patient does have some ST-T wave changes noted in the inferior leads. The only other EKG done on this patient recently was done at Central Hospital, and these records have been requested but are currently pending.

Complete chest x-ray was performed and showed the heart to be at the upper end of normal for a portable film; otherwise, no abnormalities were noted. There have been recommendations for a repeat PA and lateral film in the near future.

Cardiac enzymes showed a total CPK of 75, MB 0.7, troponin quantitative of 0.02. Comprehensive metabolic profile showed a sodium of 140, potassium 3.3, minimally elevated alkaline phosphatase level of 135. White blood cell count is slight elevated at 12,000, with no left shift present. Hemoglobin 15.1, hematocrit 44.4.

DIAGNOSIS

1. Atypical chest pain. I am concerned about the patient's prior history of coronary artery disease. I do not feel that this is a cardiac event, but will start patient on aspirin and beta blocker, as she should be on that at this time anyway. I have recommended that she follow up immediately with a primary care physician and set up a stress test. I would recommend that they also evaluate the need for a cholesterol-lowering agent and an ACE inhibitor on this individual in the very near future. Patient also did report some palpitation-like sensations with the chest tightness and we will place a Holter monitor on her at this time.

2. Mild hypokalemia. Patient was given 40 mEq of oral KCl.[5] She is to eat a banana daily for the next several days. This can be followed up by the primary care physician.

Footnotes:

1. 1.Although stated in a kind of odd way, this means the patient does have a history of cardiac problems in her family.
2. 2.Than = expression of contrast or comparison. Then = at that time or soon after that.
3. 3.It would be acceptable to edit this as 2.
4. 4.A positive Homans' sign is an early indication of deep venous thrombosis. The sign is named for John Homans (as opposed to Homan). Therefore, the possessive form is Homans' (and not Homan's).
5. 5.The abbreviation KCl stands for potassium chloride. The K and C are capped, and the l is lowercase.

SPELLING.
Determine if the following words are spelled correctly. If the spelling is correct, leave the word as it has already been entered. If the spelling is incorrect, provide the correct spelling.

1. sweeting _____

2. tibial _____

3. hypocalemea _____

4. bilateraly _____

5. rhythem _____

MULTIPLE CHOICE.

Choose the correct spelling of the term.

1. Rapid or irregular heartbeat.

   ○ palpation

   ○ pallapitation

   ○ palpitation

   ○ palpition

2. A class of drugs used to relieve stress on the heart.

   ○ beta blockers

   ○ betae blockers

   ○ betta blockers

   ○ beata blockers

3. Pertaining to the back or dorsum of the foot.

   ○ dorsel peddle

   ○ dorsel pedal

   ○ dorsal pedal

   ○ dorsal pedle

4. Abnormally rapid heartbeat.

   ○ tachacardia

   ○ tachycardia

   ○ tachacardea

   ○ tackycradia

5. An inclination to vomit.

   ○ nasea

   ○ nausea

   ○ naussea

   ○ naussia

EMERGENCY ROOM REPORT 6

HISTORY: Patient[1] is a 79-year-old male who presents today with complaints of a 3-day history of nausea and vomiting with last episode occurring last night. He recently had a TURP on July 5, 2005, here at St. Eligius Hospital. Since that period 10 days ago, he has a history of anorexia, hiccoughs,[2] and infrequent bowel movements. He has a history of anorexia.

Bowel movements include one 2 days after leaving the hospital that was small, one episode of diarrhea four days later, and then another very small, firm bowel movement today.

He has lost 12–15 pounds in the last 10 days and reports difficulty swallowing meals. The patient reports that he discontinued his pain medications the day after he got home status post his TURP, and he is currently wearing an adult diaper due to urinary incontinence following the surgery.

He has a past surgical history significant for benign prostatic hypertrophy, colon polyps, and hypertension.

He has a surgical history positive for a gastric procedure where one third of his stomach was removed and his gallbladder.

OBJECTIVE: He is 70 inches tall, weighs 168 pounds, temperature 97.7, pulse 89, respirations 20, blood pressure 128/57. Pain is 0. General: Patient is a very cooperative and pleasant 79-year-old male who is hiccoughing. HEENT: Ocular movements intact. Mucous membranes moist. Oropharynx: Clear. Cardiovascular: Regular rate and rhythm without murmurs, rubs or gallops. Pulmonary: Lungs are clear to auscultation bilaterally. GI: Abdomen is soft, nondistended, diffusely tender, which is greatest in the left lower quadrant. Bowel sounds are present in all 4 quadrants. Neuro: Nonfocal.

LABORATORY FINDINGS: CBC, CMP, and UA were performed. UA is significant for urinary tract infection.

IMAGES: KUB[3] was performed, flat and upright. The image was read as nonspecific small bowel gas, including colon was full of stool.

ASSESSMENT

1. Constipation
2. Urinary tract infection

PLAN: Ciprofloxacin 250 mg b.i.d. for 10 days. Phenergan suppository per rectum 1 every 6 hours as needed for nausea and vomiting. Magnesium citrate 1 bottle to be drunk when he gets home. Dulcolax suppository per rectum q.6 h. for constipation. The patient has also been advised to return to the emergency room if his condition worsens.

Footnotes:

1. 1.Many dictators do not dictate "the patient," but rather simply "patient." Some clients will require this be expanded out to "The patient," but many will have it simply edited as dictated.
2. 2.This is also acceptably (and maybe more frequently) edited as hiccups (no difference in meaning).
3. 3.KUB = kidney, ureter, and bladder.

MULTIPLE CHOICE.
Choose the best answer.

1. On exam the patient has moist (○ mucus, ○ mucous) membranes.

2. The patient reported one episode of (○ diarrhea, ○ diarhhea).

3. The patient has a positive history for benign (○ prosthetic, ○ prostatic) hypertrophy.

4. Following the surgery, the patient experienced urinary (○ incontence, ○ incontinence).

5. The patient has a history of (○ anorexia, ○ anorrhexia).

TRUE/FALSE.
The following terms are spelled correctly: true or false?

1. magnesium citrate

    ○ true

    ○ false

2. Phenergen

    ○ true

    ○ false

3. pulmonery

    ○ true

    ○ false

4. cardiovasclar

    ○ true

    ○ false

5. hiccough

    ○ true

    ○ false

EMERGENCY ROOM REPORT 7

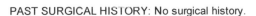

Medical Record

CHIEF COMPLAINT: Cut while playing basketball.

HISTORY OF PRESENT ILLNESS: Patient was playing basketball at around noon today. He was hit with an elbow right above his right eyebrow. After being hit with the elbow, he fell to the ground and hit the back of his head. Patient did not lose consciousness. He has no headache and there is no pain.

PAST MEDICAL HISTORY: Depression, high cholesterol, and hypercholesterolemia.

MEDICATIONS: Include Tramadol 50 mg, Tylenol 325 mg, aspirin 325 mg, paroxetine 40 mg, rabeprazole 20 mg, atorvastatin 80 mg, and naproxen 500 mg.

PAST SURGICAL HISTORY: No surgical history.

REVIEW OF SYSTEMS: No nausea, vomiting, diarrhea. No loss of consciousness. No fevers or chills. No neck pain. No abdominal pain. No chest pain. No shortness of breath.

PHYSICAL EXAMINATION: Generally, the patient is alert and oriented in no acute distress. Weight is 198, pulse 76, temperature 97.8, blood pressure 131/81, respirations are 16. Head: There is a 7-cm round hematoma in the right parietal region. There is also a 2-cm laceration above the right eyebrow that is about 2 mm deep. Pupils are equally round and reactive to light. Extraocular muscles are intact. Nasal septum is midline. There are no sores in the mouth. Mucous membranes are moist. Heart: Regular rate and rhythm without murmurs. Lungs are clear to auscultation bilaterally. Abdomen has positive bowel sounds and is soft. Neurologic: Cranial nerves are intact. Vision is 20/20. Sensation is normal in all 4 extremities. Strength is +5/5 in all 4 extremities. Reflexes are +2/4. Patient has a normal gait.

ASSESSMENT/PLAN: A 2-cm laceration above the eyebrow. Patient stated that he was sensitive to scarring. We ordered a consultation with surgical repair of the wounds by Plastic Surgery, which was performed. Patient was told to follow up in Vascular Surgery Clinic in 10 days.

SPELLING.
Determine if the following words are spelled correctly. If the spelling is correct, leave the word as it has already been entered. If the spelling is incorrect, provide the correct spelling.

1. cranial _____

2. scaring _____

3. septim _____

4. rabaprazole _____

5. naproxen _____

True/False.
Mark the following true or false.

1. The patient lost consciousness.

   ○ true

   ◉ false

2. The patient has a past medical history of depression.

   ○ true

   ○ false

3. The patient was taking naproxen 325 mg.

   ○ true

   ○ false

4. Pupils were equally round and reactive to light.

   ○ true

   ○ false

5. The patient wanted a plastic surgery consult because he was sensitive to scarring.

   ○ true

   ○ false

EMERGENCY ROOM REPORT 8

The patient is a 56-year-old gentleman. He has had myocardial infarctions times two.[1] He had a stent placed last year. He states he has not had any anginal pain[2] like he had prior to his myocardial infarctions but states that last Wednesday, after a heated argument with his son, he took a 3-mile walk. Shortly after the walk he developed some sharp chest pains, which he rated at 8/10, that lasted about 20 minutes, and apparently was helped with a nitroglycerin tablet.

Patient did report some associated shortness of breath but states he had just finished his walk. He did not have any radiating neck, jaw, arm, or back pain. Patient, as mentioned, stated that the pain was different than the discomfort associated with myocardial infarctions in the past.

OBJECTIVE FINDINGS
VITAL SIGNS: Temperature 95.9, pulse 73, respirations 20, blood pressure 116/67, weight 254 pounds.
HEART: Regular rate and rhythm without murmur.
LUNGS: Clear to auscultation bilaterally.
NECK: No JVD noted.
EXTREMITIES: No pedal edema noted.
ABDOMEN: Mildly obese, nontender, nondistended. No organomegaly. No hepatojugular reflux noted.
TRUNK: On palpation chest wall does reproduce his pain.

ED COURSE: In light of the patient's coronary artery history, we did do a full cardiac workup. He did receive an aspirin and was placed on 2 liters of O2 per nasal cannula immediately after arrival.

An EKG was performed and this showed a sinus rhythm, rate 70. No ST-T wave changes were seen. We also did a portable chest x-ray that showed no acute cardiopulmonary changes.

DIAGNOSIS: Atypical chest pain. Suspect this is chest wall in origin. There may be a certain anxiety component to it as well.

PLAN: We will set this patient up with an exercise stress test. He is to use nitroglycerin should he have recurrent chest pain. We will be glad to see him on an as-needed basis.

Footnotes:

1. 1.Also acceptably edited as x2 or x 2, although the general preference is to not put a space between the x and 2.
2. 2.Angina refers to a spasmodic, choking, or suffocative pain, and often is referring to angina pectoris—a paroxysmal thoracic pain.

MULTIPLE CHOICE.
Choose the best answer.

1. Patient had a (○ stent, ○ stint) placed last year.
2. The patient's abdomen is nontender and (○ nondisdended, ○ nondistended).
3. The patient's chest pain was somewhat relieved with a (○ nitroglyceran, ○ nitroglycerin) tablet.
4. Upon arrival, the patient received oxygen per nasal (○ cannula, ○ canulla).
5. The patient's chest pain is considered (○ atypical, ○ atypicle).

MULTIPLE CHOICE.

Choose the correct spelling of the term.

1. Listening to sounds within the body.

   ○ asculatation

   ○ auscultation

   ○ ausultation

   ○ ausciltation

2. Affecting both the heart and the lungs.

   ○ cardiapulmonary

   ○ cardiapulminary

   ○ cardiopulminary

   ○ cardiopulmonary

3. Inhaling and exhaling.

   ○ resperation

   ○ resperashun

   ○ respireration

   ○ respiration

4. Relating to the middle muscular layer of the heart wall.

   ○ miocardiale

   ○ myocardial

   ○ myocardiale

   ○ myocardyle

5. Of or relating to the right and left sides of the body.

   ○ bilaterally

   ○ bilatrally

   ○ billateraly

   ○ bilateraly

EMERGENCY ROOM REPORT 9

HISTORY OF PRESENT ILLNESS: This 57-year-old white male comes in with pain in the lower-left abdomen rated a 2 on a scale of 1 to 10, last Sunday, Monday, and Tuesday, not today. He has had a similar pain of the penis head with spasms. He has had a collection of cerumen in the right and left ear with a hearing impairment for the last 4 years. He has had a sinus infection almost always. He has had a chest infection, questionable mucus, for the last 6 months, coughing up mucus, etc. He has shortness of breath with this.

He has a feeling of congestion, question if it is water or pain around the heart for the last 2 months. It lasts for approximately 1 second or less. He has had filmy eyes. No history of asthma. He has had some wheezing. He is around smokers. He has a history of hemorrhoids. He has arthritis pains in the left wrist, lower back, and right wrist. He has had an outbreak of clear fluid of vesicles of the right cheek, right buttock, and on his back. The right cheek had a vesicle 6 months ago, which he scratched, and he has kept scratching it since that time. It does not really itch, but he keeps peeling the hematoma off. There may have been a black-green vesicle fluid within this, 6 months ago.

He had a black stool 1 week ago for 1 week in mid April that was continuous, and none since that time. He has not been able to keep any food in his stomach but he is always hungry. He is not having any emesis.

He has had a history of alcohol abuse. He quit alcohol 20 years ago and remains off alcohol. He has used AA at times. His best friends are AA people. He has had intermittent thoughts of suicidal ideation, which has been very deep and he may have had alcoholic parents. Approximately 2 weeks ago his father died, and the patient re-experienced that he has had problems with his own 2 children pretty deeply throughout his life. He has no active suicidal ideation now.

PHYSICAL EXAM:[1] VITAL SIGNS show 176, 97, 59, 20, 138/89.[2] HEENT shows no sinus tenderness. The THROAT is normal appearing. The NECK is supple without any adenopathy or thyromegaly. The spine was nontender to palpation. Murphy's sign was absent for the kidneys. The HEART shows regular rhythm and rate. The LUNGS are clear with decreased breath sounds bilaterally. ABDOMEN shows normoactive bowel sounds, nontender, without any mass or hepatosplenomegaly. EXTREMITIES do not show any edema. SKIN shows hematomas of the right cheek and several of the back that appear as scratch marks. I see no vesicles or other types of lesions right now.

DIAGNOSIS

1. Dermatitis
2. Ears show bilateral cerumen impaction
3. Depressive disorder

PLAN

1. Hydrocortisone cream t.i.d. to the rash sparingly
2. Debrox otic drops 2 drops twice a day for 2 weeks
3. See back in 2 weeks or return sooner if any problems

I offered to refer him to see the staff psychiatrist today, he declined this. He did promise to come back and see me if he has any doubts or any thoughts of suicide developing. He will come to the emergency room if this occurs evenings, weekends, or nights and see his PCP if it is during the day.

Footnotes:

1. 1.This PE was edited using a specific format likely requested by the client. Typically, when ALL CAPS are used in a subheading, a colon and/or left justification are also used. Again, this is an account-specific format.
2. 2.This is a different way to express the vital signs; the dictator does not dictate the measurement parameters—temperature, weight, etc. In this example, the information is likely weight 176, temperature 97, pulse rate 59, respiratory rate 20, and blood pressure 138/89. You would not add these unless account instructions require you add them (and unless you are completely sure what the measurements are).

FILL IN THE BLANK.

Using the word(s) in the box, enter the appropriate term in the space provided.

1. Patient is diagnosed with _____ disorder.

2. Patient currently has no suicidal _____.

3. Patient is prescribed _____ drops for his ears.

4. Neck exam reveals no _____ or thyromegaly.

5. Patient complains of _____ impaction in both ears.

adenopathy
cerumen
depressive
ideation
otic

MATCHING.

Match the exam phrase to the appropriate anatomy, body system, or PE subheading.

1. ____ Regular rate and rhythm.   A. skin

2. ____ Nontender without hepatosplenomegaly.   B. heart

3. ____ No vesicles or lesions.   C. neck

4. ____ Blood pressure.   D. vital signs

5. ____ Supple.   E. abdomen

UNIT 3

Physical Medicine

PHYSICAL MEDICINE – INTRODUCTION

Physical medicine and rehabilitation is the branch of medicine that covers the ongoing treatment for physical problems, such as severely broken bones, torn ligaments, knee and hip replacements, rehab for spinal injuries, postsurgical rehab, and similar conditions. The words *physical medicine* may conjure up images of an elderly person in an after-stroke condition, perhaps receiving speech therapy, learning to walk and properly hold utensils again. Many people (likely either you or someone you know) have had some form of physical therapy during their lifetime: after a car accident, an illness, a major surgery, or even for carpal tunnel syndrome—an ailment all too common to professions in which repetitive motion is an inciting factor.

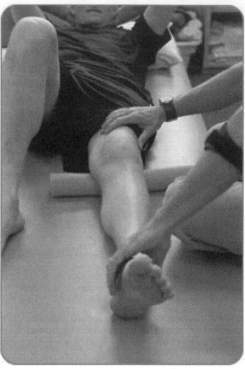

Physical medicine and rehabilitation (often called PM&R) assists the patient in restoring functionality due to a physical disability. The subspecialties and specialties of physical therapy, occupational therapy, orthopedics, sports medicine, and chiropractics all fall under the general umbrella of physical medicine. Also included in PM&R are all of the maneuvers, positions, anatomical planes, and assistive devices associated with physical medicine. You may hear the word **physiatrist** in reference to this branch of medicine, which is properly spelled physiatrist, but pronounced as fiz-eye-uh-trist. A physiatrist practices in PM&R.

Common conditions that are treated by physiatrists include (but are certainly not limited to):

- amputation
- spinal cord injury
- sports injury
- stroke
- musculoskeletal pain syndromes such as low back pain and fibromyalgia
- traumatic brain injury

Physical medicine can be part of a hospital course, as well as outpatient treatment for prolonged periods of time. There is also physical therapy and rehab for internal structures, primarily reconditioning the heart, as in a patient status post a heart attack. As with the previous chapters, the editing of physical medicine reports is usually done as a separate department within a hospital. There are also physical therapy and rehabilitation centers whose primary concern is some type of physical therapy, either for admitted patients or on an outpatient basis.

PHYSICAL MEDICINE LANGUAGE

As you are introduced to PM&R, you will notice a language of its own developing. Shortened forms of words and abbreviations are abundant in this specialty, as you will see. The reason for this has to do with the spectrum of conditions that physiatrists treat: spinal cord injuries, cardiac rehabilitation (rehab), neck and back pain, ergonomic education to prevent or heal injury, pain management, hospice care, sports injury, amputee conditioning and training, and so many more "subcategories." At the helm and intertwined with so many of these subcategories is the specialty of orthopedics.

In reviewing this terminology, you will run across familiar and unfamiliar terms, which will only expand upon your existing knowledge base. In addition to the abbreviations and shortened forms of words, there will be some definitions provided that you are likely to find in the PM&R language. You may hear a dictator state, "The patient was ordered to OT where ADLs will be assessed to determine if a FWW is needed." There are a plethora of physiatrist-specific books and websites available—these are extensive due to the layers of subspecialties and variety of treatment modalities. The language lists in this unit cover some of the more common terms one can expect to hear or see when editing for the vast specialty that is physical medicine and rehabilitation.

PHYSICAL MEDICINE LANGUAGE WORKSHOP

Physical therapists, and physiatrists in general, will refer to the position of a structure in relationship to another. An example would be the kidneys being superior to (above) the urinary bladder. The following table indicates some of the anatomical positions you might expect to come across in the field of physical medicine and rehabilitation and what they mean.

Anatomic Positions/Directional Terms

Term	Meaning
cranial	toward the head
caudal	toward the feet
medial	toward the middle
lateral	toward/from the side
proximal	toward the limb's attachment
distal	toward the fingers/toes
superior	above
inferior	below
anterior	toward the front
posterior	toward the back
peripheral	toward the surface
palmar	toward the palm of the hand
plantar	toward the sole of the foot

A patient visiting an orthopedist or one who is involved in a physical therapy/occupational therapy protocol ordered by a physiatrist is subject to a bevy of tests and maneuvers. In addition, signs of anomaly are sought in order to properly identify treatment and course of action for the patient. Some of the terminology you can expect to hear may sound like someone's surname, which is precisely the derivative of many of these diagnostic tools and exercises. Please note that the preference is to drop the possessive form of the term, so that Tinel's sign, named after French neurologist Jules Tinel, is preferred as "Tinel sign." Account specifics may dictate otherwise. Other than repetition and time, there is no "set in stone" way to learn these. Familiarity breeds retention.

The website WhoNamedIt.com is a helpful eponym resource.

Tests, Maneuvers, and Signs

Test/Maneuver/Sign	Usage/Evaluation
External rotation test	ankle
Anterior drawer test	ankle
Tinel sign	wrist
Yergason test	shoulder
Waddell test	lumbar spine
French Horn shoulder test	shoulder
Quadriceps femoris muscle angle	knee
Straight leg raise	lumbar spine
Costoclavicular maneuver	evaluate thoracic outlet syndrome/costoclavicular syndrome
Probe-to-bone test	evaluate osteomyelitis/diabetic foot ulcers
Galeazzi sign	hip disorder evaluation
Phalen maneuver	carpal tunnel syndrome evaluation
Lachman test	anterior cruciate ligament rupture (ACL)
Trendelenburg symptom	hip evaluation (not to be confused with trendelenburg anatomic position)
Talar tilt (inversion stress test)	for lateral ankle sprains

Abbreviations are abundant in medical transcription editing, and it is no different in the PM&R world. Below is a listing of some of those most commonly used abbreviations. Manuals and textbooks have been written which encompass all of the abbreviations used in physiatry, so the list below is but a smattering of the prevalent ones. Remember also that these are the most common physical medicine-related expansions. Most, if not all, of these abbreviations will have additional correct expansions not PM&R related (for example, ER = emergency room).

Common PT Abbreviations

Abbreviation	Expansion
AE	above elbow
AKA	above-knee amputation
AFO	ankle-foot orthosis or orthotic
BKA	below-knee amputation
CPM	continuous passive motion
DJD	degenerative joint disease
DF	dorsiflexion
ER	external rotation
HOB	head of bed
ITB	iliotibial band
KAFO	knee-ankle-foot orthosis
MMT	manual muscle test
NWB	nonweightbearing
PROM	passive range of motion
SD	shoulder disarticulation
SLR	straight-leg raise
TTWB	toe touch weightbearing
TKA	total knee arthroplasty
WNL	within normal limits

During the recovery process and as part of daily usage, the patient may be trained and instructed in use of assistive devices and aids. A resource book, such as *Stedman's Medical and Surgical Equipment*, will serve as a valuable resource to your library and/or electronic version of resources. Below is a listing of some of the commonly heard assistive and training device abbreviations and terms.

Assistive and Training Devices

Assistive Device/Term	Translation/Used For
FWW	front-wheel walker
QC	quad cane
SBQC	small base quad cane
PUW	pick-up walker
Spica splint	thumb
O & P	orthotics and prosthetics
C-cane	straight cane with curved handle
hemiwalker	quad cane/walker combo
brace	knee, leg, arm
moldable insert	lumbosacral
immobilizer	knee
Jobst boot (brand)	foot
Endo-MATE endotracheal tube holder	ENT device
Stryker (brand)	hip, knee, shoulder implants
Allocraft C-ring	cervical spacer used in diskectomy and fusion surgery of the spine
wound VAC	vacuum-assisted closure for wounds
grab bars	for bathroom safety
Hoyer lift	assistance in lifting bed/chair ridden patients
Vehicle lifts	assisting patients in wheelchairs
Aspen cervical collar (brand)	cervical stabilization

Finally, no section on physical therapy and rehabilitative medicine would be complete without some terms about the conditions themselves. Physiatrists treat symptoms from cranium to plantar arch and then some. With this in mind, here are some conditions that require the assistance, aid, and/or expertise of experts in this field.

Conditions	Translation/Used For
cavus foot	high arch
temporomandibular joint (TMJ)	jaw/head
plantar fasciitis	foot
epicondylitis	tennis elbow/swimmer's elbow
rickets	osteomalacia in children
claudication	limping, lameness
hypotonia	muscular tonicity loss
kyphosis	humpback
de Quervain disease	wrist
gout	metabolic disease of uric acid crystals in tissues
Heberden nodes	bony swelling around joint margins
tenosynovitis	overuse of tendons from trauma, overuse
dysphagia	trouble with eating or swallowing
hemiplegia	paralysis on one side of the body
cystoid macular edema	swelling of macula of eye resulting from injury, surgery, or disease
diabetic retinopathy	affecting patients with diabetes
burn therapy	for patients with severe burns (grafting, whirlpool)
post pregnancy scarring	pelvic floor rehab is used for this, including kegel exercises
osteoarthritis	may require hip replacement (arthroplasty)

REVIEW: PHYSICAL MEDICINE LANGUAGE

MULTIPLE CHOICE.
Choose the correct expansion of the abbreviation.

1. Wound VAC – wound vacuum-(○ assisting, ○ assisted) closure

2. O & P – orthotics & (○ prosthetics, ○ programming)

3. HOB – (○ headboard, ○ head) of bed

4. SLR – straight (○ ligament, ○ leg) raise

5. FWW – (○ framed, ○ front)-wheel walker

SPELLING.
Determine if the following words are spelled correctly. If the spelling is correct, leave the word as it has already been entered. If the spelling is incorrect, provide the correct spelling.

1. Galeazzi _____

2. periphral _____

3. dorsyflexion _____

4. Yirgason _____

5. caudul _____

6. tenosinovitis _____

7. immobilizer _____

8. chostoclavicular _____

9. dysarticulation _____

10. Lachman _____

MATCHING.
Match the correct term to the definition.

1. ____ Toward the middle.

2. ____ Toward the sole of the foot.

3. ____ Below.

4. ____ Toward the back.

5. ____ Toward the surface.

6. ____ Toward the head.

7. ____ Toward the front.

8. ____ Toward the palm of the hand.

9. ____ Toward/from the side.

10. ____ Toward the feet.

A. peripheral

B. medial

C. lateral

D. inferior

E. anterior

F. cranial

G. plantar

H. caudal

I. palmar

J. posterior

TRUE/FALSE.
Mark the following true or false.

1. Rickets is a form of chickenpox.

    ○ true

    ○ false

2. A hoyer lift assists patients only in the hospital.

    ○ true

    ○ false

3. WNL stands for within negative limits.

    ○ true

    ○ false

4. If a patient has TMJ disorder, they might see an ENT doctor.

    ○ true

    ○ false

5. BKA is a below-knee assistive device.

    ○ true

    ○ false

PHYSICAL MEDICINE REPORTS

The terminology involved in physical medicine includes many orthopedic terms. Rehabilitation doctors treat nerves, muscles, bones, and brains—decreasing pain and restoring function. Some maneuvers, positions, and other terms are unique to physical therapy transcription editing. If you are unsure of terms as you move through the physical medicine reports, make sure to look them up or come back to the language workshop. (You may also find it helpful to review the Muscles unit in the Anatomy and Disease module.)

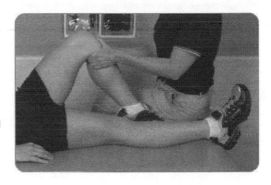

To review, most of the reports you will be exposed to in this Physical Medicine unit will be consultation and progress note reports. Multispecialty clinics will commonly have a physical medicine representation through pain management, physical therapy, and occupational therapy departments.

PHYSICAL MEDICINE REPORT 1 – CONSULTATION

DIAGNOSIS: Left thumb sprain.

SUBJECTIVE: The patient is a 51-year-old teacher. She injured her thumb when she fell at work, apparently landing on her thumb. The thumb was initially casted for 3 days and then splinted for 2–3 weeks. It was then left free for 2 weeks. Then it was recasted again until [DATE]. Patient reports the doctors were not sure if there was a fracture or injured ligament. She reports that x-rays were done but no other studies.

She describes pain on the ulnar side of the IP and MCP joints[1] of the thumb. She has pain upon motion, but no pain at rest. She presently is not taking any medications and has not previously injured the thumb. She is working full duty with a 20-pound lifting restriction.

OBJECTIVE: The thumb appeared mildly swollen. Range of motion: MCP right 0/50, left 0/50. IP right 0/86, left 0/70. Abduction: Right 0/45, left 0/40. Other than the thumb, range of motion was within normal limits. Patient is right-hand dominant. Grip strength was measured using the Jaymar dynamometer placed at the second setting: Right 60 pounds, left 41 pounds. Lateral pinch: Right 13 pounds, left 11 pounds. Three point pinch: Right 12 pounds, left 6 pounds. Thumb/index pinch: Right 11.5 pounds, left 7 pounds. Patient reports no abnormal sensation. Since the cast was removed on February 5, she reports the thumb is somewhat tender, but she has been using it for everyday light activities.

ASSESSMENT/RECOMMENDATIONS: Objective findings are consistent with a left thumb injury, possibly a sprain of the ulnar collateral ligament. Range of motion and strength are diminished on the left compared to the right.

LONG TERM GOALS:[2]

1. Normal strength and range of motion will be restored.
2. Prevention of reinjury to the thumb.
3. Resume normal work duties including lifting heavy objects.

SHORT TERM GOALS:

1. Increase grip strength by 10 pounds within 2 weeks.
2. Increase pinch strength by 2 pounds within 2 weeks.
3. Restore full range of motion within 2 weeks.
4. Patient will be instructed in joint protection and body mechanics to prevent reinjury of the thumb during this stage of healing.

SHORT TERM PLAN:

1. Ultrasound treatments.
2. Use of heat and cold modalities to control pain and edema.
3. Initiate range of motion exercises.
4. Initiate strengthening exercises.
5. Initiate education in joint protection and body mechanics.

Footnotes:

1. 1. IP and MCP are the interphalangeal and metacarpophalangeal joints, respectively.
2. 2. You will notice that physical medicine reports include a variety of headings and subheadings not typically seen in other specialties. Occasionally the formatting will include the use of tables of information as well. We will not be including any tables in our physical medicine examples. Some tables are built into the report template (meaning the headings and tables are prepopulated and the information filled in as it is dictated).

MULTIPLE CHOICE.

Choose the correct spelling of the term.

1. Relating to the ulna.
   - ulnaer
   - ulner
   - ulnare
   - ulnar

2. Moving away from central axis of body.
   - abduction
   - adbuction
   - adduction
   - aduction

3. Situated at or extending to the side.
   - latral
   - laterel
   - lateral
   - latteral

4. Thick short innermost digit of the hand.
   - thum
   - thumb
   - thunb
   - thumd

5. Measuring instrument designed to measure power.
   - dynamameter
   - dynammometer
   - dynamometer
   - danymometer

TRUE/FALSE.
Mark the following true or false.

1. Other than the thumb, the patient's range of motion is within normal limits.

    ○ true

    ○ false

2. The patient is to use cold and no heat to control the swelling.

    ○ true

    ○ false

3. Ultrasound treatments are part of this patient's short term plan.

    ○ true

    ○ false

4. The patient is 57 years old.

    ○ true

    ○ false

5. This patient's thumb is currently casted.

    ○ true

    ○ false

PHYSICAL MEDICINE REPORT 2 – CONSULTATION

DIAGNOSIS: Status post left tib-fib[1] fracture.

Thank you for referring Frank Lee[2] to our clinic. He was seen on December 21, 2005, for evaluation and treatment of his right[3] lower extremity as you requested.

SUMMARY OF PHYSICAL THERAPY FINDINGS

SUBJECTIVE: The patient reports injuring left lower extremity when walking down a driveway and slipping and falling on ice. He suffered fractures of the left distal tibia and proximal fibula. He was casted with an above-the-knee long leg cast for approximately 6 weeks and then fitted into an ankle-hinged walking plastic brace which did not include the knee. He is presently ambulating 40% weightbear,[4] which is to progress to full weightbear in the following 2 weeks. Presently he reports he is pain free and denies any tingling or numbness in the left lower extremity.

OBJECTIVE SIGNIFICANT FINDINGS:

1. Gait: Ambulates to clinic with crutches approximately 40% weightbearing left lower extremity with plastic hinged ankle brace, left lower extremity.
2. Active range of motion: Left knee 123 degrees flexion. Right knee is equal to 135 degrees flexion. Left knee 5 degrees extensor lag. Left ankle dorsiflexion 0 degrees to 30 degrees plantar flexion. Right ankle dorsiflexion 15 degrees to 50 degrees plantar flexion. Left ankle eversion 20 degrees to 5 degrees inversion. Right ankle eversion 40 degrees to 45 degrees inversion.
3. Passive range of motion: Left knee 0 degrees to 135 degrees flexion with pain, patellar with tightness at end range flexion. Left ankle 5 degrees dorsiflexion to 35 degrees plantar flexion with stretch of the calf. Left ankle eversion 25 degrees to 10 degrees inversion pain free.
4. Manual muscle test: Right ankle strong and nonpainful. Right knee strong and pain free.
5. Left knee evaluation: Negative ligaments, negative McMurray test.
6. Left ankle evaluation: Nonspecific tenderness, left ankle ligaments and no laxity of ligaments noted.

ASSESSMENT: Ten weeks status post left tib-fib fracture with swelling, decreased range of motion of the left knee and ankle, general atrophy secondary to disuse.

The following goals were developed in conjunction with Frank.

SHORT TERM GOALS (six treatments):

1. Decrease swelling.
2. Increase active range of motion of the left ankle and left knee.

SHORT TERM PLAN: Physical therapy 3 times per week for interferential stimulation to decrease swelling and progressive range of motion exercise to restore left knee and ankle joint mobility with gentle progressive strengthening as tolerated.

LONG TERM GOALS (sixteen treatments):

1. Ambulation without assistive device.
2. Strength left knee and ankle 5/5 pain free.
3. Squat and stairs independently without difficulty.

LONG TERM PLAN: Left total lower extremity strengthening program to include flexibility, closed chain, proprioceptive, and balance activities.

Thank you for allowing us to see the patient. I will keep you informed of his progress. If you have any questions or comments, please feel free to contact me.

Footnotes:

1. 1.This is short for tibia-fibula.
2. 2.This is a made up name. The name has been changed for HIPAA compliance.
3. 3.The dictator states "right" leg here, but everywhere else it appears the left leg is the injured leg. It would be a really good idea to flag the dictation here for clarification.
4. 4.The term *weightbear*, as it sounds, means to bear weight. Your spell checker will not likely approve of it being spelled as one word. However, this is one of those words that is spelled as one word frequently in medical transcription editing. It would not be incorrect, however, to spell this as two words.

SPELLING.

Determine if the following words are spelled correctly. If the spelling is correct, leave the word as it has already been entered. If the spelling is incorrect, provide the correct spelling.

1. ambalation _____

2. inversion _____

3. dorsaflexion _____

4. fibila _____

5. numness _____

True/False.

Mark the following true or false.

1. He was casted with a below-the-knee long leg cast.

    ○ true

    ○ false

2. He reports that he is pain free but has some tingling and numbness in the lower extremity.

    ○ true

    ○ false

3. His short-term goals include 6 treatments.

    ○ true

    ○ false

4. He is eleven weeks status post left tib-fib fracture.

    ○ true

    ○ false

5. He would like a long-term goal of 5/5 left knee and ankle strength pain free.

    ○ true

    ○ false

PHYSICAL MEDICINE REPORT 3 – DISCHARGE SUMMARY

REFERRING PHYSICIAN: John Jones, MD.

DIAGNOSIS: Multiple sclerosis.

DATE OF ONSET: Approximately 8 years ago.

SUBJECTIVE: This patient is a 33-year-old female who states that she began to have problems with her balance approximately 8 years ago. At that time it was diagnosed that her condition was multiple sclerosis. Her complaints consist of fatiguing easily after prolonged activity and losing her balance during ambulation easily. When the patient was last seen on October 23, she stated she felt like she was walking better with fewer balance problems and stated she wanted to continue these exercises on her own at home without ongoing physical therapy visits.

OBJECTIVE: This patient was seen for a total of 6 physical therapy treatments beginning on August 14, and ending on October 23, 2007. These treatments consisted of balance and coordination exercises to improve balance and coordination of the lower extremities during weightbearing and ambulation and also included gait training, emphasizing knee flexion and dorsiflexion of the feet. When the patient was last seen on October 23, it was noted that her knee flexion and ankle dorsiflexion had improved significantly, which helped to normalize her gait. In addition, she was able to perform a sit-to-stand activity with greater ease. Her standing balance reactions are improved. She is independent with a home exercise program to continue these coordination and balance activities.

ASSESSMENT: This patient responded quite well to physical therapy to improve the balance and coordination during weightbearing activities. She is independent with a home exercise program, and it is felt that she will continue to practice these coordination and balance activities at home. She is very pleased with the progress she has made performing these activities. Since she has achieved her physical therapy goals outlined in the objective section of this form, we are discharging her from physical therapy.

Thank you again for this referral to our facility. If I can be of any help with any questions or concerns you may have, please feel free to give me a call.

SPELLING.
Determine if the following words are spelled correctly. If the spelling is correct, leave the word as it has already been entered. If the spelling is incorrect, provide the correct spelling.

1. weightbearing _____

2. therape _____

3. flexioun _____

4. coordination _____

5. balence _____

MULTIPLE CHOICE.
Choose the best answer.

1. The patient has been diagnosed with multiple (○ sclerosis, ○ sclerosus).

2. Patient (○ fatigues, ○ fatiges) easily after prolonged activity.

3. Patient's (○ gate, ○ gait) has normalized with exercise.

4. The patient now performs sit-to-stand activities with greater (○ ease, ○ eaze).

5. Patient loses balance during (○ ambalation, ○ ambulation).

PHYSICAL MEDICINE REPORT 4 – CONSULTATION

DIAGNOSIS: Right shoulder pain.

Thank you for referring B.J. Smith to our clinic. He was seen on March 11, 2006, for evaluation and treatment of his right shoulder as you requested.

SUMMARY OF PHYSICAL THERAPY FINDINGS

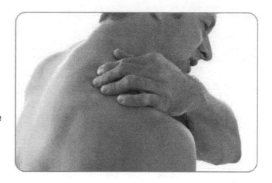

SUBJECTIVE: The patient reports chronic right shoulder pain which has not been significantly improved with physical therapy and cortisone injections. He reports that he has persistent popping and clicking in the right shoulder and has increased pain of the right shoulder when sleeping on his right side. He reports he is unable to throw or do any significant lifting with the right upper extremity due to increased pain. He reports he has intermittent tingling and numbness in his right fifth and fourth[1] fingers associated with severe increases of pain. He reports that rest decreases the pain, and any activity of the right shoulder increases the pain. He reports that the shoulder feels extremely fatigued with use.

SIGNIFICANT OBJECTIVE FINDINGS:

1. Posture: Right shoulder and scapula are elevated. Cervical is within normal limits.[2]
2. Active range of motion: Right shoulder is within normal limits, pain free. Overpressure increases pain in external rotation.
3. Resistive tests: Pain produced with external rotation and abduction, although all muscle groups show a strength of 5/5.
4. Special tests: Pain produced with end range shoulder adduction with elbow extended with applied overpressure.
5. Palpation: Tenderness of right teres minor musculature and insertion tenderness of right supraspinatus muscle belly and insertion.

ASSESSMENT: Chronic right shoulder pain with possible rotator cuff and/or labrum dysfunction.

The following goals were developed in conjunction with B.J.

SHORT TERM GOALS (six treatments):

1. Decrease irritability of the right teres minor and supraspinatus muscle and tendon.
2. Pain-free resistive external rotation and abduction.
3. Decrease guarding and increase flexibility of the right shoulder to allow for symmetrical posture of upper trapezius and left scapula.

SHORT TERM PLAN: Physical therapy 3 times per week for ultrasound, friction massage, heat and cold pack to reduce tenderness, gentle range of motion and flexibility exercise program to improve muscle balance throughout the right shoulder girdle musculature. Physician primarily wants a resting program for the right rotator cuff.

LONG TERM GOALS (twelve treatments):

1. Sleep right side lying down without discomfort, measured by subjective report.
2. Throw a softball and lift in excess of 200 pounds bilateral upper extremities without discomfort, measured by subjective report.

LONG TERM PLAN: Progressive right shoulder strengthening, especially rotator cuff, as physician allows. Challenge functional activities and recreational activities as physician allows.

Thank you for allowing us to see the patient. I will keep you informed of his progress. If you have any questions or comments, please feel free to contact me.

Footnotes:

1. 1.It would be perfectly acceptable to edit this as 5th and 4th. Ordinals can be written out or edited as ordinals (except with dates; it is not typically acceptable to edit March 11th, even if dictated that way).
2. 2.Cervical is an adjective meaning (in this context) of or relating to the neck. Its use here doesn't completely make sense—cervical WHAT? It is likely the dictator is referring to the cervical spine being within normal limits. A flag might be warranted for clarification. It would be inappropriate to insert a word or guess at the meaning. Transcription editing as dictated and leaving a flag for clarification is the best practice for this situation.

True/False.
Mark the following true or false.

1. The patient has reported constant tingling and numbness in his right fifth and fourth fingers.

   ○ true

   ○ false

2. His left shoulder and scapula are elevated.

   ○ true

   ○ false

3. The physical therapist's assessment was that the patient might have a possible rotator cuff and/or labrum dysfunction.

   ○ true

   ○ false

4. The patient will begin with physical therapy 6 times per week.

   ○ true

   ○ false

5. The patient would like to be able to throw a softball and lift in excess of 200 pounds without discomfort.

   ○ true

   ○ false

SPELLING.
Determine if the following words are spelled correctly. If the spelling is correct, leave the word as it has already been entered. If the spelling is incorrect, provide the correct spelling.

1. cortisone _____

2. intermitent _____

3. labruum _____

4. resistative _____

5. teras minor _____

PHYSICAL MEDICINE REPORT 5 – CONSULTATION

DIAGNOSIS: Bilateral wrist and forearm overuse syndrome.

SUBJECTIVE: At this time patient reports she is experiencing intermittent pain, especially when not wearing her splints. She describes this pain as shooting pains that extend through her volar forearm, right arm greater than left. She states that she has some numbness in her ulnar digits of the right hand. Patient reports that her pain is worse when she goes without her splints at work, and also when she puts weight on her right hand, as in heavy lifting tests. She states that her pain is relieved somewhat by taking hot baths. At this time she states she is taking ibuprofen and no other medication. She denies ever having any similar problems before or receiving other therapy. At this time she wears splints provided by her physician while at work.

OBJECTIVE: Patient is a 42-year-old female who works as a mail services supervisor. She states that in November she was performing mail sorting tasks and typing and began to experience bilateral wrist pain which she describes as an aching. She reports that this progressed into volar forearm pain bilaterally. At this time patient is referred by Dr. Syd Hansen for OT evaluation and treatment.

WORK HISTORY: Patient has worked at this job for the last 4 years. She states that she is working presently full time with the following restrictions: Patient is to work no more than 8 hours a day, no repetitive hand grasping activities, no repetitive wrist or elbow motion, and no keyboard work.

VERBAL JOB ANALYSIS: Patient reports her job includes sorting mail manually, typing tasks, 10-key operation, and unloading supplies from trucks. She states that she normally works 10-hour days. Patient reports that approximately 1 hour out of her day is spent sitting, and the rest is standing or walking tasks. She states that she must lift a maximum weight of approximately 60 pounds. She reports these are trays of mail which she can carry less full if necessary. She states that an average lift weight is about 30 pounds and states that probably 40% of her job requires lifting. She states most lifting is performed from waist to overhead height. She states she also must do some pushing and pulling with a 4-wheel cart which she estimates weighs up to 150 pounds when completely loaded. She states she does some carrying tasks with about 30 pounds for 20–30 feet in distance. Her goal for employment is to return to her previous duties without any pain.

Upper extremity range of motion and function: Patient's upper extremity active range of motion is within normal limits throughout. Patient was negative for Tinel sign. The patient, when performing Phalen test[1], reported numbness and tingling in ulnar digits bilaterally. Patient reports she had EMGs[2] done on both upper extremities approximately 2 weeks ago.

Upon palpation, therapist was able to locate tenderness in flexor muscle bellies on the volar surface of both forearms. Patient also displays tenderness at lateral epicondyles bilaterally. The patient reports no increased pain with resisted wrist flexion or extension at this time. There is no swelling apparent visually.

Sensation: Formal sensory evaluation was not performed on this date. Patient reports no sensory disturbances, with the exception of ulnar digits, especially on right hand, feeling colder than the other digits at times. Therapist will perform formal sensory evaluation next session.

Strength: Grip: 65 pounds right, 74 pounds left (dominant). Lateral pinch: 16 pounds right, 16 pounds left. Two point pinch: 10 pounds left, 14 pounds right. Three point pinch: 17 pounds right, 18 pounds left.[3]

ASSESSMENT: At this time it appears that patient would benefit from OT 3 times a week to decrease symptomatology in both upper extremities and to increase functional tolerance to work and ADL tasks.[4]

SHORT TERM GOALS:

1. Patient will report decrease in pain level in both upper extremities.
2. Patient will demonstrate correct postures of daily living in work-simulated tasks in clinic.
3. Patient will correctly perform home exercise program in clinic and follow through at home.

LONG TERM GOALS: Patient will return to work to previous duties without restrictions and without increased symptomatology.

PLAN: Occupational therapy 3 times a week to achieve the above stated goals.

SHORT TERM PLANS:

1. Introduce patient to fluidotherapy and ultrasound.
2. Initiate home exercise program.
3. Initiate postures of daily living and body mechanics training.

LONG TERM PLANS: Patient will perform exercise program on BTE[5] to increase bilateral upper extremity strength and endurance for work tasks.

Thank you for allowing us to see the patient. I will keep you informed of her progress. If you have any questions or comments, please feel free to contact me.

Footnotes:

1. 1.If you are unsure what is involved in a Tinel and/or Phalen test, now is a great time to look these tests up online.
2. 2.EMG = electromyogram, a graphic representation of the electric currents associated with muscular action.
3. 3.This strength testing information is the type of information that is presented frequently in a table format. As you can likely imagine, it would be easier to read in a table format.
4. 4.ADL = activities of daily living.
5. 5.BTE stands for Baltimore Therapeutic Equipment, which is a work simulator.

MULTIPLE CHOICE.

Choose the correct spelling of the term.

1. Position or arrangement of the body and its limbs.

   ○ postur

   ○ posture

   ○ postore

   ○ pustoure

2. Denoting the palm of the hand or sole of the foot.

   ○ vollar

   ○ voller

   ○ volar

   ○ voler

3. A test for carpal tunnel syndrome in which both hands are held tightly palmarflexed, opposite to a prayer position.

   ○ Tinel

   ○ Phalen

   ○ Tinnel

   ○ Phalin

4. A projection on a bone above a condyle.

   ○ epacondyle

   ○ eppicondyle

   ○ epecondyle

   ○ epicondyle

5. Sensation of tingling or "pins and needles."

   ○ Tinel

   ○ Phalen

   ○ Tinnel

   ○ Phalin

TRUE/FALSE.
The following terms are spelled correctly: true or false?

1. symptomatology

   ○ true

   ○ false

2. ocupational

   ○ true

   ○ false

3. sensary

   ○ true

   ○ false

4. tingling

   ○ true

   ○ false

5. treatement

   ○ true

   ○ false

SUBJECTIVE: This patient reported that on August 8, he ran over his foot with a pallet jack. He was diagnosed as having a fracture in the foot and a possible avulsed tendon of the extensor hallucis longus. When his cast was removed at the beginning of September, complaints consisted of pain with weightbearing into the fourth metatarsal and lack of motion secondary to extreme edema in the right foot. Currently this patient relates that his foot is feeling much better, and he has significantly increased his active range of motion in the right ankle. However, he still complains of moderate pain in the foot upon weightbearing and prolonged ambulation.

OBJECTIVE: This patient was seen for a total of 14 physical therapy treatments beginning in September 2007 and ending in December 2007. These treatments consisted of whirlpool with active range of motion exercises to the right foot, aerobic stationary bike, Stairmaster, balance and proprioception exercises to the right ankle, joint mobilization, and home exercises for strengthening of the right ankle joint complex. As of December 17, active range of motion of the right ankle included 18 degrees of dorsiflexion, 27 degrees of plantar flexion, 36 degrees of inversion, and 9 degrees of eversion. A figure-of-eight girth measurement around the right ankle was recorded to be 53 cm. This patient was instructed on home exercises to be performed for strengthening of the right joint complex. Accessory mobility of this joint was normal to slightly hypermobile.[1] This office was contacted on December 19 by Dr. James Williams when he stated that this patient should discontinue physical therapy visits at this clinic and continue strengthening exercises at home on his own.

ASSESSMENT: This patient was responding extremely well to physical therapy. However, his progress has been slow the past couple of weeks. Since he has been discharged from physical therapy by his physician, we are therefore discharging him from our active files.

Footnotes:

1. 1.Hypermobility is excessive mobility or free movement.

SPELLING.

Determine if the following words are spelled correctly. If the spelling is correct, leave the word as it has already been entered. If the spelling is incorrect, provide the correct spelling.

1. hypermobeal _____

2. avulsed _____

3. gurth _____

4. aerobic _____

5. plantar _____

MULTIPLE CHOICE.

Choose the best answer.

1. Treatments consisted of whirlpool with active range of (○ motion, ● flexion) exercises.

2. Active range of motion of the right ankle included 36 degrees of (● eversion, ● inversion).

3. Patient had a possible avulsed tendon of the extensor (● pollicis, ● hallucis) longus.

4. Accessory (● motility, ● mobility) of the joint was mostly normal.

5. Patient complains of moderate (● ankle, ● foot) pain upon prolonged ambulation.

PHYSICAL MEDICINE REPORT 7 – CONSULTATION

DIAGNOSIS: Left knee injury.

Thank you for referring the patient to our clinic. He was seen on May 8 for evaluation and treatment of his left lower extremity, as you requested.

SUMMARY OF PHYSICAL THERAPY FINDINGS

SUBJECTIVE: The patient reports hitting his left inner lower knee against several objects, such as a wall and concrete. He developed a lump in the left medial tibial plateau with severe swelling and ecchymosis over the next day. He is presently applying medication and ice, although he has progressive pain and edema with worsening since the injury. He denies previous left knee problems.

SIGNIFICANT OBJECTIVE FINDINGS

1. Gait: Patient ambulates to clinic without assistive device with severe limp, left lower extremity. Left lower extremity is maintained in abduction and external rotation position to prevent knee flexion or ankle dorsiflexion.
2. Observation: He has approximately a 4 in x 3-1/2[1] in lump noted in the left medial tibial plateau that is hard in nature and red in color. He has severe bruising that extends from approximately 2 inches suprapatellar, medial aspect greater than lateral, which extends all the way down through the calf to the ankle and into the foot.
3. Circumference: Ankle: 11 inches left and 10-1/2 inches right, swelling. Calf: 17 inches left and 16 inches, swelling. Knee: 16-1/2 inches left and 15-1/2 inches right, swelling.
4. Passive range of motion: Left knee with minus 5 degrees[2] extension to 90 degrees flexion. Left ankle dorsiflexion to neutral plantar flexion to 20 degrees. Inversion to 10 degrees, eversion to 10 degrees.
5. Active range of motion: Left knee 15 degrees extensor lag to 90 degrees flexion. Left ankle minimal movement. Left knee and ankle range of motion limited secondary to pain.
6. Strength: Left ankle 5/5. Left knee not tested due to severe tenderness.
7. Sensation: Diminished throughout left lower extremity.
8. Palpation: Tenderness to entire left lower leg.

ASSESSMENT: Contusion, left medial tibia, with severe swelling and ecchymosis throughout left lower leg with decreased range of motion, ankle and knee.

Footnotes:

1. 1. If the measurement was metric (mm or cm), you would say 3.5 instead of 3-1/2. It is generally preferred not to use fractions with metric units of measurement.
2. 2. This could be edited as -5 degrees.

SPELLING.
Determine if the following words are spelled correctly. If the spelling is correct, leave the word as it has already been entered. If the spelling is incorrect, provide the correct spelling.

1. contusion _____
2. aproximately _____
3. extremety _____
4. inversion _____
5. bruiseing _____

True/False.
Mark the following true or false.

1. The patient had a right knee injury.

   ○ true

   ○ false

2. The patient ambulated to the clinic with a severe limp.

   ○ true

   ○ false

3. The lump in the knee was soft in nature and red in color.

   ○ true

   ○ false

4. There has been progressive pain and worsening edema since the injury.

   ○ true

   ○ false

5. No ecchymosis was present in the lower leg.

   ○ true

   ○ false

PHYSICAL MEDICINE REPORT 8 – CONSULTATION

DIAGNOSIS: Cervical sprain.[1]

SUBJECTIVE: Patient reports that she was in a rear-ended motor vehicle accident in November. She sustained a straining type of injury to her neck, as well as a traumatic crush to her right hand. Presently the right side of her neck is quite painful and tender to touch. The patient has recently undergone reconstructive hand surgery in December. As a result of the hand surgery, some of the cervical evaluation was deferred.

SUMMARY OF SIGNIFICANT FINDINGS

1. Pain with range of motion at the end of side bend left and rotation left.
2. Decreased segmental mobility at level C1-C2 and C2-C3[2] on the right.
3. Positive TMJ[3] involvement on the right side. It is to be noted that the patient is being treated by her dentist for the TMJ issue, so it will not be addressed in therapy.

ASSESSMENT: This patient should respond to a short course of therapy to reduce muscle spasm and pain, as well as increase mobility.

Goals are as follows.

SHORT TERM GOALS (5 visits)

1. Pain free[4] range of motion within normal limits.
2. Increase segmental mobility to within normal limits.
3. Patient will show correct execution with home exercise program.

SHORT TERM PLAN

1. Ultrasound, heat, soft tissue mobilization.
2. Joint mobilization.
3. Range of motion exercises.

LONG TERM GOALS (10–12 visits)

1. Normal range of motion.
2. Normal segmental mobility.

Footnotes:

1. 1. You should always put a period at the end of a statement of declarative information. Just because this is only 2 words doesn't mean it is okay to leave off the period.
2. 2. This is also acceptably edited as C1-2 and C2-3. It is not necessary (although perfectly acceptable) to repeat the same letter before the second vertebra when expressing the space between two vertebrae.
3. 3. TMJ = temporomandibular joint.
4. 4. You may have noticed that sometimes this is edited as pain-free range of motion and sometimes pain free range of motion. The industry trend is away from using hyphens when the meaning is clear. There is acceptable variation to how this information can be presented accurately.

Mark the following true or false.

1. The patient's long term goals are projected to take 10–12 visits.

   ○ true

   ◉ false

2. The patient has not yet undergone surgery for injuries suffered in the automobile collision.

   ◉ true

   ○ false

3. The patient was injured when her vehicle rear-ended another vehicle.

   ◉ true

   ○ false

4. The patient's short term goals include proper execution of home exercise program.

   ◉ true

   ○ false

5. The patient's TMJ will be treated with joint mobilization exercises in PT.

   ◉ true

   ○ false

MULTIPLE CHOICE.
Choose the best answer.

1. This patient should respond to a short (○ coarse, ○ course) of therapy.

2. The patient is being treated by her dentist for her (○ temporomandiblar, ○ temporomandibular) joint issues.

3. The patient sustained a (○ tramatic, ○ traumatic) crush to her hand.

4. Goal is to increase (○ segmental, ○ segamental) mobility to within normal limits.

5. The patient's short term plan includes soft tissue (○ immobilization, ○ mobilization).

PHYSICAL MEDICINE REPORT 9 – CONSULTATION

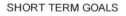

DIAGNOSIS: Possible carpal tunnel syndrome and lateral epicondylitis on the right.

SUBJECTIVE: The patient is a 27-year-old employee who works as a proof support specialist. She reports that she has pain in the volar forearm and wrist, and the long and ring fingers swell and go numb at times. She describes the pain as an aching pain. She reports that the numbness and swelling occur mostly at night and early in the morning. After awaking and moving the hands the symptoms subside. She is taking ibuprofen. She has been wearing a Futuro wrist brace at work and at night.

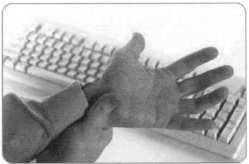

OBJECTIVE: Range of motion was within normal limits. Five part grip strength was measured using a Jaymar dynamometer: Right hand 60 pounds, left hand 51 pounds. Lateral pinch: Right 16 pounds, left 15 pounds. Three point: Right 9.5 pounds, left 9. Thumb/index: Right 11 pounds, left 10 pounds.

SPECIAL TESTS: Phalen test was administered. After 1 minute in this position she reported that her index, middle, and ring fingers "felt fat and heavy," but there was no pain. Finkelstein test was negative. Tinel test was negative at the elbow but positive at the right wrist. There was some mild tenderness at the medial epicondyle, but no reports of discomfort at the lateral epicondyle. Manual muscle testing was performed, and strength of all muscle groups of the right hand was felt to be normal. A sensory test was not done today.

WORK HISTORY: The patient has been employed as a proof support specialist for 6 months. She is presently working full duty with the only restriction being that she wear her brace at work. Her job involves sitting and working at a keyboard. She reports that there are time pressures and productivity quotas, and employees do take mandatory breaks to stretch every hour and a half. She feels that her workstation fits well and is properly adjusted.

> Carpal tunnel syndrome is a serious concern for medical transcription editors. Preventative measures, such as an ergonomic workstation including appropriate desk height and ergonomic keyboard, as well as wrist splints, stretching, and targeted exercises, will go a long way in preventing or alleviating wrist pain for MEs. To find out more about CTS go to www.ncbi.nlm.nih.gov /pubmedhealth/PMH0001469/ .

ASSESSMENT/RECOMMENDATIONS: Objective findings today are somewhat inconsistent with the referring diagnosis of carpal tunnel syndrome and left lateral epicondylitis. Grip and pinch strengths were normal with slightly higher strength on the right side compared to the left. With CTS it would be expected that grip and pinch strengths might be lower on the affected side. There was no tenderness upon palpation and no Tinel sign at the lateral epicondyle, but the patient did report tenderness of the medial epicondyle. Phalen test was atypical for carpal tunnel syndrome, in that the ring finger was involved and there were no reports of symptoms affecting the thumb. Patient does not present today with clear symptoms of carpal tunnel syndrome or lateral epicondylitis. There were no objective findings of any abnormality today. She did report subjective findings during the Phalen test and subjective reports of pain.

PLAN: Five more occupational therapy sessions will be scheduled per Dr. Dana Stowe's order. Emphasis will be placed on education for prevention of repetitive motion injuries. Ultrasound treatments will be initiated.

SHORT TERM GOALS

1. Patient will continue full work duties without complaints of pain that interfere with her work.
2. Grip and pinch strengths will remain within normal limits.
3. Patient will demonstrate understanding of joint protection techniques during exercises in the clinic.

SHORT TERM PLAN: Five ultrasound treatments, progressive resistive exercises, instruction in joint protection techniques, use of heat and cold modalities as needed to control pain symptoms.

Unscramble.
Unscramble the underlined word in each term below and fill in the complete word at the end.

1. npaehl test _____

2. leint sign _____

3. cnpacoouilta therapy _____

4. Jaymar treemayonmd _____

5. itnekleifns test _____

6. parcal tunnel syndrome _____

7. turouf wrist brace_____

8. lateral condylitisepi_____

UNIT 4

Radiology

RADIOLOGY – INTRODUCTION

When you think of radiology, you likely think of the term *x-ray*, and you probably even imagine a picture of a bone or a chalky white silhouette of the lungs. Radiology, of course, is more than that. Radiology is the branch of medicine dealing with radioactive substances and radiant energy and with the diagnosis and treatment of disease by both roentgen rays and ultrasound radiations.

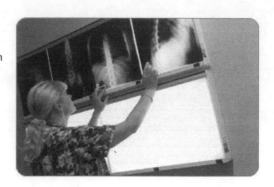

Radiology as a medical specialty is an umbrella term covering a variety of subdivisions. For our purposes we will break radiology into two main types:

1. Diagnostic Radiology – The interpretation of images of the human body to aid in the diagnosis of disease.

2. Therapeutic Radiology – The use of radiation for treatment of disease.

Depending on who you work for as an MTE, you can do a wide variety of diagnostic radiographic examinations or a very limited number. For example, if you work for a small hospital, clinic, or doctor's office it is possible that you will edit x-ray reports, but only those that can be performed in such an institution: chest x-rays, back x-rays, and orthopedic x-rays. However, a larger hospital will likely have an extensive radiology department that may encompass a multitude of different types of radiologic examinations to include all the simple x-rays, but also MRIs, CTs, voiding cystourethrograms, mammograms, GI studies, nuclear studies, cholangiograms, obstetrical ultrasounds, and many others. In fact, some hospitals have a separate transcription editing department for the radiology. The vocabulary for simple bone and chest x-rays is easier and more limited than that used for the more complex types of examinations. Chest x-rays that are performed outside of a large hospital on an outpatient basis will usually be less complex than those done on a patient in a hospital.

Typically—and this is only typically, mind you—therapeutic radiology reports are edited specifically by radiology transcription editors. We have included therapeutic radiology reports in this unit in an effort to expose you to as much radiology as possible.

RADIOLOGY LANGUAGE

Did you ever have a sense that something was going on or about to happen in your life, yet you just couldn't pinpoint what it was or how it would happen? A premonition, perhaps? Radiology is a premonition, of sorts, brought into clarity/focus. X-rays, as the basic energy source of study in the radiology field, are generally a starting point for diagnosis of condition, anomaly, and/or disease. However, the study of radiology and nuclear medicine has so expansively grown, that x-rays are but one of the many tools physicians use in their diagnostic summation.

Within this unit, we will be exploring several types of radiology, terms you can expect to hear on reports, and the contrast media agents used in the tests themselves.

Radiology transcription editors often have additional training and specialize in the language that accompanies this field. In fact, entire word books are devoted to the topic, including *Stedman's Radiology Words*.

If you have not yet started to keep a word list, now is a REALLY great time to start. A word list is just that—a list of words. These may be unfamiliar (new to you) words or phrases or words for which you want the exact spelling. Sometimes word lists even include definitions. Compiling and maintaining your own word list is a great learning tool, not to mention a fabulously valuable resource in the pursuit of accurate productive medical transcription editing.

RADIOLOGY LANGUAGE WORKSHOP

Depending on the type of diagnostic test being performed and the area of focus, the patient is required to assume a position. Some of the different anatomic patient positions you can expect to hear on radiologic reports are found in the first chart below. In addition to the way the patient is positioned, the radiologist uses anatomic planes. Some of the anatomical planes of the body follow.

Patient Positions

Patient Position	Description
supine	Patient lying on the back, face up.
prone	Patient lying on the stomach, face down.
lateral decubitus	Patient lying down on side, x-ray beam positioned horizontally.
recumbent	Patient lying down, either prone or supine.
flexion	Patient bending a specific part of the body.
extension	Patient lengthens or straightens a flexed limb.
inversion	Patient turning inward.
posterior-anterior (PA view)	Most common chest x-ray view. The x-ray goes from a source placed posteriorly to a detector placed anteriorly.
anteroposterior view (AP)	The x-ray goes from a source placed anteriorly to a detector placed posteriorly.
left lateral view	The x-ray goes from a source located to right of patient to a detector located to the left of the patient.
oblique view	The x-rays will travel in a slanted direction at an angle stemming from the perpendicular plane. Regions normally hidden in PA or AP view will appear in oblique views.

Anatomical Planes

Anatomic Plane	Description
frontal (coronal)	Vertical plane divides the body into anterior and posterior. The PA view of a chest x-ray uses the frontal plane.
sagittal (lateral)	Unequal right and left sides.
midsagittal (median)	Right and left halves. Lateral chest x-ray (side-to-side) uses the sagittal plane.
transverse (horizontal)	Upper (superior) and lower (inferior) portions. CT scan uses the transverse plane.
longitudinal plane	Cuts along the long (longitudinal) axis of the body.
transpyloric plane	This is a transverse plane named so because it should cross over the pylorus of the stomach.
midcoronal (midaxillary) plane	A longitudinal plane which cuts through the head and body along the coronal suture of head and extends down through the body.

Within all fields of medicine, there remains a constant language. As you know by now, at the heart of this language are prefixes, suffixes, root words/combining forms, and medical terminology itself. The following table showcases some of the vernacular commonly used in radiology.

Radiology Word Parts

Term	Word Part	Meaning
-opaque	suffix	obscure, as in radiopaque
-lucent	suffix	to shine, as in translucent
cine-	prefix	movement, as in cineradiogram
echo-	prefix	repeated sound, as in echocardiogram
-graphy	suffix	process of recording, as in ultrasonography
son/o	root word	sound, as in sonogram
tom/o	root word	to cut, as in tomography
is/o	root word	same, as in radioisotope
-gram	suffix	record, as in cardiogram
ultra-	prefix	beyond, as in ultrasonogram
roentgen/o	root word	x-ray, as in roentgenology
fluor/o	root word	luminous, as in fluoroscopic
scint/i	root word	spark, as in scintigraphy (note the spelling is with an "i")
viv/o	root word	life, as in in vivo
vitr/o	root word	glass, as in in vitro

And finally, the following list of radiology abbreviations should serve as a review, as you have already been exposed to radiology abbreviations in the Mastering Medical Language module.

Common Radiology Abbreviations

Abbreviation	Meaning
AP	anteroposterior
AP/PA	anteroposterior/posteroanterior
Ba	barium
BE	barium enema
C1-7	cervical vertebrae 1-7
CAT scan	computerized axial tomography scan
CMG	cystometrogram
CT	computed tomography
DICOM	digital image communication in medicine (meaning transmission between imaging devices)
EEG	electroencephalogram
ERCP	endoscopic retrograde cholangiopancreatography
GI	gastrointestinal (usually upper GI—the area examined)
HIDA	hydroxyiminodiacetic acid
IVP	intravenous pyelogram
KUB	kidneys, ureters, bladder
L1-5	lumbar vertebrae 1-5
LS	lumbosacral (films)
MRI	magnetic resonance imaging
MUGA	multiple gated acquisition
OCG	oral cholecystogram
PA	posteroanterior
PACS	picture archival and communications system
PET	positron emission tomography
T1-12	thoracic spine 1-12
UGI	upper gastrointestinal (series)
US or U/S	ultrasound
VCUG	voiding cystourethrogram

REVIEW: RADIOLOGY LANGUAGE

MULTIPLE CHOICE.
Choose the best answer.

1. Frontal indicates a (⊙ vertical, ⊙ horizontal) plane that divides the body into anterior and posterior.

2. An EEG is an (⊙ electroencephalogram, ⊙ echocardiogram).

3. KUB is a scan of the kidneys, (⊙ ureters, ⊙ urethra), and bladder.

4. Sagittal view means of (⊙ equal, ⊙ unequal) right and left sides.

5. A voiding (⊙ cystourethrogram, ⊙ cystourography) is abbreviated VCUG.

SPELLING.
Determine if the following words are spelled correctly. If the spelling is correct, leave the word as it has already been entered. If the spelling is incorrect, provide the correct spelling.

1. proctosigmoidoscopy _____   2. pyelogram _____

3. rentgenology _____   4. sagital _____

5. lumbasacral _____

TRUE/FALSE.
Mark the following true or false.

1. The prefix cine- means picture.

    ⊙ true

    ⊙ false

2. A vertical plane that divides the body into anterior and posterior is transpyloric.

    ⊙ true

    ⊙ false

3. In a recumbent position, the patient must lie down supine.

    ⊙ true

    ⊙ false

4. The transpyloric plane cuts down the long axis of the body.

    ⊙ true

    ⊙ false

5. PET stands for positional emissions tomography.

    ⊙ true

    ⊙ false

MATCHING.

Match the correct term to the definition.

1. ____ X-rays that travel in a slanted direction.

2. ____ X-rays that go from anterior source to posteriorly placed detector.

3. ____ Patient lying on back.

4. ____ Patient lying on stomach.

5. ____ Straightening a flexed limb.

6. ____ Bending a specific body part.

7. ____ Common chest x-ray view.

8. ____ Patient turns inward.

9. ____ X-ray taken from source to right of patient to detector to left of patient.

10. ____ Patient lying on side with x-ray beam horizontal.

A. extension

B. oblique

C. left lateral view

D. lateral decubitus

E. AP view

F. flexion

G. supine

H. prone

I. PA view

J. inversion

MULTIPLE CHOICE.

Choose the correct expansion for the abbreviation.

1. MUGA
   - ○ multiple gated acquisition
   - ○ multiple gated aquisition
   - ○ multiple gaded acquisition
   - ○ multiple gated aquisition

2. HIDA
   - ○ hexaminodiacetic acid
   - ○ hepatoaminodiacetic acid
   - ○ hydroxyiminodiacetic iminodiacetic acid
   - ○ hydroxyiminodiacetic acid

3. SPECT
   - ○ single-photon emision computed tomography
   - ○ single-photon emission compuded tomography
   - ○ single-photon emission computed tommography
   - ○ single-photon emission computed tomography

4. CT
   - ○ computer topography
   - ○ computer tomography
   - ○ computed tomography
   - ○ computed topography

5. PA
   - ○ posteranterior
   - ○ posteroanteror
   - ○ posteroanterior
   - ○ posterioranterior

DIAGNOSTIC RADIOLOGY REPORTS

Diagnostic radiology involves the interpretation of images of the human body to aid in the diagnosis of disease. Simple x-rays (or radiographs) are a large part of this field. However, as you are well aware, there are other procedures, such as CTs, MRIs, ultrasounds, mammograms, and nuclear scans, that fall under the category of radiology but are not simple (or plain) x-rays as you may understand them. As a clinical medicine transcription editor, you will likely be exposed to radiology reports in some way, shape, or form. Radiology clinical practices have their own in-house transcription editors or outsource to a service. In smaller hospitals, Radiology will be part of the medical records transcription editing department, and in larger hospitals, radiology departments will have their own transcription editors. There are also independent radiological reading institutions, where radiology specialists read various x-rays for smaller clinics or doctor's offices. This is because x-ray reports are required to be read by a trained radiology specialist.

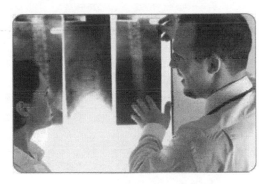

Additionally, you may type radiologic terms, in essence a mini-radiology report, in discharge summaries, patient clinic notes, or various other report types, as indications in an operation report or as part of the history, laboratory data, or hospital course.

As we touched on in the introduction to this unit, diagnostic radiology covers a wide variety of subtypes and can be divided by anatomic location and in some cases by method. The report types we will be studying in this unit include:

Make sure to read the footnotes, when applicable, in the reports as they are full of definitions, transcription editing tips, verification hints, and thought processes for accurate documentation.

- Bone X-Rays
- Chest X-Rays
- Abdominal X-Rays
- MRI
- CT Scans
- Contrast Studies
- Ultrasounds
- Mammograms

While these reports do not begin to cover all types of diagnostic radiology, the groupings will give you thorough exposure to the most common types of radiology reports. Often the x-ray reports are very short, and to that end we have multiple x-ray reports per report page. You will, of course, come across more radiology files in the practicum modules of this training program.

This unit is quite long, but it is filled with important information for a thorough understanding of radiology. Take your time. Work on one grouping at a time. Take frequent breaks. If it wasn't important, we wouldn't include it.

BONE X-RAY REPORTS 1–3

CLINICAL HISTORY

1. Assault.
2. Crepitus[1] of the left jaw.

FACIAL BONES: No fracture is seen. The sinuses appear clear. The right frontal sinus appears hypoplastic.[2] No fractures of the mandible are seen, although the coronoid processes and TMJs are not completely evaluated, and a subtle fracture could be missed.

IMPRESSION: No fractures. Given the patient's history, TMJ views may be useful if indicated.

Footnotes:

1. 1.Crepitus has the same meaning as crepitation and crepitance—a crackling or grating noise from the joints, skin, or lungs.
2. 2.If you aren't sure what this word means, break it down. The prefix *hypo-* means below normal and *-plasia* means development or formation; put them together and you get underdeveloped.

CLINICAL HISTORY: Twisted ankle while walking, with a history of fracture of the same foot and ankle twice before.

RIGHT ANKLE: There is soft tissue swelling overlying the lateral malleolus. A small accessory ossicle[1] or old avulsion fracture is seen adjacent to the tip of the lateral malleolus. There is no evidence for acute fracture. There is fusion of the tibial growth plate with incomplete fusion of the fibular growth plate.

IMPRESSION: No evidence of a fracture or dislocation.

Footnotes:

1. 1.Aren't sure what an ossicle is? Look it up!

CLINICAL HISTORY: Follow up fracture of the right wrist.

RIGHT WRIST: Bony sclerosis and periosteal new bone is present just proximal to the metaphysis of the distal radius, consistent with healing fracture. The growth plate of the distal radius appears intact. Alignment on the AP view appears normal, but there is approximately 15 degrees of dorsal angulation of the distal radial articular surface.

IMPRESSION: Healing distal radius fracture with dorsal angulation.

SPELLING.
Determine if the following words are spelled correctly. If the spelling is correct, leave the word as it has already been entered. If the spelling is incorrect, provide the correct spelling.

1. dorsel _____

2. malleolus _____

3. fusoin _____

4. metyphsis _____

5. avulsion _____

MATCHING.
Match the correct term to the definition.

1. ____ Shaped like a crow's beak, hooked or curved.

2. ____ A small bone.

3. ____ A crackling or grating noise, often coming from the joints or lungs.

4. ____ Angular deformity to a fractured bone.

5. ____ Situated around bone.

A. ossicle

B. angulation

C. coronoid

D. crepitus

E. periosteal

BONE X-RAY REPORTS 4–6

CLINICAL HISTORY: Low back pain and left hip pain times 2–3 weeks. No trauma, and no neurologic deficit.

LUMBOSACRAL SPINE SERIES: Bones are mildly osteopenic.[1] Degenerative changes are noted throughout the lumbosacral spine, most marked at T11-12 and T2-3. There is mild anterolisthesis of L3 with respect to L2. Facet sclerosis is present at L5-S1 posteriorly. No definite osteoblastic lesions are seen within the lumbar spine, but if metastatic disease is a concern, bone scan is more sensitive. Incidentally noted is an atheromatous plaquing[2] of the abdominal aorta, whose lumen measures 3 cm. Multiple collections of barium are seen within diverticula.

AP PELVIS: Postoperative clips and sutures are present in the true pelvis. Hips are within normal limits for age. Sacroiliac joints are unremarkable. No definite lytic or osteoblastic[3] processes are seen. Incidental note is made of phleboliths in the pelvis.

IMPRESSION

1. Degenerative changes of the lumbosacral spine, most marked at L2-3.
2. No acute bony findings.

Footnotes:

1. 1.Again, if you break down the word into its parts: osteo- means bone and -penia means deficiency; osteopenic is the adjectival form of osteopenia.
2. 2.Atheromatous plaquing is when there is fibrous deposit accumulating on the artery lining.
3. 3.You will also hear this dictated as simply "blastic."

CLINICAL HISTORY: A 57-year-old man with history of numbness in the left leg.

LUMBOSACRAL SPINE AND PELVIS: No bony destructive lesions seen. Disk height and vertebral body alignment are normal. Diffuse idiopathic skeletal hyperostosis of the lumbar spine is seen. Pelvis: Normal.

IMPRESSION

1. Diffuse idiopathic skeletal hyperostosis[1] of lumbar spine without significant degenerative disk[2] changes.

Footnotes:

1. 1.This is commonly dictated as DISH. Note also, this was edited with a 1 in this list, and this is most likely because it was dictated that way and the client prefers it this way. Typically, however, a 1 is not edited (even when dictated) unless there is also at least a 2.
2. 2.This can be acceptably edited as disc as well.

CLINICAL HISTORY: This 38-year-old male suffered multiple blunt traumas to head and thorax, causing pneumomediastinum.

CERVICAL SPINE: Vertebral body heights and disk spaces appear preserved. There is air dissecting through the prevertebral soft tissues, consistent with dissection from pneumomediastinum, as given in the patient's history. No increase in the amount of prevertebral soft tissue is seen. No evidence of fracture or subluxation. Neural foramina are patent bilaterally.

IMPRESSION: Streaky air in the prevertebral soft tissues. This is consistent with dissection from pneumomediastinum as given in the patient's history.

SPELLING.
Determine if the following words are spelled correctly. If the spelling is correct, leave the word as it has already been entered. If the spelling is incorrect, provide the correct spelling.

1. thorax _____

2. prevretebral _____

3. sacrailiac _____

4. osteoblastic _____

5. placquing _____

MULTIPLE CHOICE.
Choose the correct spelling of the term.

1. The condition in which air is present in the mediastinum.

   ○ pneumomediastinum

   ○ pneumomediastum

   ○ pneumediastinum

   ○ pneumomediumstina

2. A partial dislocation of a joint or organ.

   ○ subluxion

   ○ sublaxation

   ○ subluxation

   ○ subluxition

3. DISH

   ○ diffuse idiosyncric skeletal hyperostosis

   ○ diffuse idiopathic skeletal hypernecrosis

   ○ deficiency idiopathic skeletal hyperostosis

   ○ diffuse idiopathic skeletal hyperostosis

4. A calcification or stone within a vein.

   ○ phlebilith

   ○ phlebalith

   ○ phlebolith

   ○ phlebelith

5. Small bulging sacs pushing outward from the colon wall.

   ○ divreticula

   ○ diverticula

   ○ diverticuler

   ○ diverticulam

BONE X-RAY REPORTS 7–9

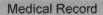

CLINICAL HISTORY: A 62-year-old with multiple myeloma and spinal cord compression with radiation therapy.

SKELETAL SURVEY: Please note that only the AP pelvis and lateral skull films are submitted for review. Lateral skull films show two lytic lesions, one in the high parietal and one in the frontal region. Old films from June 2005 show these two areas to be present at that time, without significant interval change.

AP PELVIS: Shows evidence for cortical erosion in the left aspect of L4. No definite lytic lesions are seen in the pelvis or hips, although a 2- to 3-cm lucency[1] in the right iliac bone laterally may represent a lytic lesion or perhaps overlying bowel gas. Extensive calcification is seen in the iliac vessels bilaterally. There is a tube overlying the pelvis in the midline, perhaps in the patient's rectum or in the bladder. Degenerative changes are also noted in the lumbosacral spine.

IMPRESSION

1. Lytic lesions in the skull, unchanged from June 2005.
2. Lytic lesion in the left aspect of L4.
3. Skeletal survey incomplete. Only the AP pelvis and lateral skull film were available for interpretation.

Footnotes:

1. 1.A lucency is something that has a softly bright appearance or is marked by clarity or transparency.

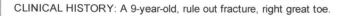

CLINICAL HISTORY: A 9-year-old, rule out fracture, right great toe.

RIGHT GREAT TOE SERIES: There is a small linear lucency noted along the distal portion of the proximal phalanx of the first toe. There is apparent resorption[1] of the tufts of the distal phalanges.

IMPRESSION

1. Low probability of a fracture of proximal phalanx of the first toe, although with tenderness at this site, recommend followup films.
2. Resorption of distal phalangeal tufts, may be normal variant, but is also seen in systemic disease. Clinical correlation required.

Footnotes:

1. <u>1.</u>Resorption means just like what it sounds like—the assimilation of substances previously produced by the body back into the body.

CLINICAL HISTORY: Preop right carpal tunnel syndrome.

RIGHT HAND: Degenerative changes are present at the second DIP and fourth and fifth PIP joints, consisting of joint space loss, osteophyte formation, and subcortical cysts. The appearance is most consistent with erosive osteoarthritis. Some milder degenerative changes are present at the first CMC joint. Soft tissue prominence adjacent to the IP joints consistent with Heberden's and Bouchard's nodes.[1] Carpal tunnel view of the wrist shows no abnormality.

IMPRESSION: As above.

Footnotes:

1. 1. You will note that sometimes the proper medical names have the possessive form, as Heberden's and Bouchard's. A client will specify whether to leave or drop possessive forms eponyms. Without specific instruction it is acceptable to do these either way. We have left some of them in place to reflect the realities of MTE and variations in style that are nonetheless acceptable.

SPELLING.
Determine if the following words are spelled correctly. If the spelling is correct, leave the word as it has already been entered. If the spelling is incorrect, provide the correct spelling.

1. osteoarthritis _____

2. pariatal _____

3. phalanx _____

4. osteophite _____

5. luccency _____

MULTIPLE CHOICE.
Choose the best answer.

1. PIP stands for proximal (○ interphalangeal, ○ introphalangeal).

2. A lesion in which a cell membrane has ruptured is said to be (○ lytec, ○ lytic).

3. CMC stands for (○ carpometacarpal, ○ carpametacarpal).

4. The term (○ phalangeal, ○ phalangial) means relating to a finger bone.

5. Bony swellings in the finger joints are referred to as (○ Heberdan's, ○ Heberden's) nodes.

CHEST X-RAY REPORTS 1–3

CLINICAL HISTORY: Recent onset of SOB[1] on mild exertion.

PA AND LATERAL CHEST: Comparison is made to the exam of February 2006. Cardiac size appears to have increased mildly. Overall cardiac size is at the upper limit of normal to mildly enlarged. Pulmonary vessels are normal. No infiltrates are present. Multiple bilateral healed rib fractures again noted.

IMPRESSION

1. Apparent mild increase in cardiac size since previous exam.
2. Otherwise stable.

Footnotes:

1. 1.SOB = shortness of breath.

CLINICAL HISTORY: Prior esophageal carcinoma, rule out lung mets[1] or effusions.

PA AND LATERAL CHEST: The patient's previous exams have been removed from the department and are not available for comparison. Heart and pulmonary vessels are normal in size. Apical, pleural, and parenchymal scarring noted bilaterally. No pulmonary infiltrates. No effusions noted. No significant bony abnormalities.

IMPRESSION

1. Apical, pleural, parenchymal scarring, otherwise unremarkable. No radiographic evidence for metastatic disease to the chest.

Footnotes:

1. 1.Mets is short or slang for metastases.

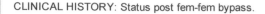
CLINICAL HISTORY: Status post fem-fem bypass.

AP PORTABLE CHEST: Comparison is made to a series of films dating back to November 2006, with the most recent on February 13, 2007. The endotracheal tube is unchanged in position, with tip 3 cm above the carina. The tip is deviating toward the right. Again noted is a nasogastric tube, which has been advanced since the most recent film, and is probably within the stomach below the level of the film. There is a left subclavian catheter, unchanged in position, with tip in superior vena cava. The diffuse pulmonary infiltrate is similar to that noted on the exam of January 21, 2007. It appears somewhat worse in this exam. However, there is a difference in positioning of the patient on these previous exams, which may partially account for the findings. The previously noted right internal jugular catheter sheath has been removed. Heart is within normal limits in size and unchanged. Central pulmonary vessels appear prominent.

IMPRESSION

1. Borderline low position of endotracheal tube.
2. Findings consistent with noncardiogenic pulmonary edema or adult respiratory distress syndrome. Cannot exclude superimposed pneumonia. Appears somewhat worse since exam in January. Patient's most recent films were not available for comparison.

SPELLING.

Determine if the following words are spelled correctly. If the spelling is correct, leave the word as it has already been entered. If the spelling is incorrect, provide the correct spelling.

1. nasagastric _____

2. apecal _____

3. pleural _____

4. abnormalities _____

5. bilatral _____

MULTIPLE CHOICE.

Choose the best answer.

1. X-ray reveals parenchymal (○ scarring, ○ scaring) bilaterally.

2. Examination revealed no (○ effusions, ○ affusions).

3. Central pulmonary vessels appear (○ prominant, ○ prominent).

4. There are no pulmonary (○ infiltrates, ○ infitrates) noted.

5. Examination cannot exclude (○ pnemonia, ○ pneumonia).

CHEST X-RAY REPORTS 4–6

CLINICAL HISTORY: Testis[1] tumor. Routine followup.

PA AND LATERAL CHEST: No previous films are available for comparison. Films have just been returned for interpretation nearly 1 year later. Heart and pulmonary vessels are normal in size. There is a large osteophyte at the left lateral aspect of the lower thoracic vertebral bodies. A 3 mm density is present in the right upper chest, probable granuloma. Lungs are clear. Bones are unremarkable.

IMPRESSION: No radiographic evidence of metastatic disease.

Footnotes:

1. 1.A testis is one of the two male reproductive glands (the pair is referred to as testes).

CLINICAL HISTORY: Withheld.

PA AND LATERAL CHEST: There are postoperative changes of a right thoracotomy with volume loss, suggesting a lobectomy. Several ill-defined, lobular, pleural base densities are noted in the left chest, probably pleural plaques. Heart and pulmonary vessels are normal in size. Calcified granulomata noted in the left apex. The patient's previous films could not be located.

IMPRESSION: Postoperative chest with findings of pleural plaques and old granulomatous disease. It is important that these films be compared to the patient's prior films if they can be located.[1]

Footnotes:

1. 1.X-rays are commonly taken as comparison films, to note changes (good or bad) in or resolution of issues.

CLINICAL HISTORY: Repair of tetralogy of Fallot.[1]

FINDINGS: Moderate cardiomegaly unchanged since November 2006, but the heart is larger since February 2006. The left cardiac border in the region of the pulmonary artery tract is prominent, suggesting pulmonary outflow hypertrophy or left atrial enlargement. In favor of left atrial enlargement is also some widening of the carinal angle.[2] This does raise the possibility of early left ventricular failure, but there is no pulmonary edema and no acute infiltrates.

IMPRESSION: Cardiomegaly, worse since February 2006, but unchanged since November 2006. Status post correction of tetralogy of Fallot. Also notes removal of sternal sutures since November.

Footnotes:

1. 1.A tetralogy of Fallot is a congenital heart defect.
2. 2.This is said a little awkwardly, but the meaning is clear—the finding of a widening carinal angle supports the suggestion of left atrial enlargement.

SPELLING.
Determine if the following words are spelled correctly. If the spelling is correct, leave the word as it has already been entered. If the spelling is incorrect, provide the correct spelling.

1. falot _____

2. hypertrophy _____

3. tetrology _____

4. thoracotomy _____

5. granulamata _____

MATCHING.
Match the correct term to the definition.

1. ____ Passing into or through by permeating.

2. ____ Abnormally enlarged heart.

3. ____ A bony abnormal outgrowth.

4. ____ Excessive accumulation of fluid in tissue.

5. ____ Tumor caused by infection or inflammation.

A. osteophyte

B. edema

C. granuloma

D. cardiomegaly

E. infiltration

CHEST X-RAY REPORTS 7–9

CLINICAL HISTORY: Post PICC line[1] placement within the left cephalic vein.

PORTABLE CHEST: Comparison is made with the study performed earlier in the day, case #8664365701. A left peripheral venous catheter is seen within the medial soft tissues of the left arm. The most medial extent of the catheter is seen at the level of the glenoid fossa. The rest of the examination is otherwise unchanged.

IMPRESSION: Left PICC visualized to the level of the glenoid fossa. Since this catheter is relatively radiopaque, recommend instillation of a small amount of contrast to assure the catheter tip position prior to initiating intravenous therapy.

Footnotes:

1. 1.PICC stands for peripherally inserted central catheter. This is also acceptably edited as PIC line.

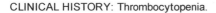

CLINICAL HISTORY: Thrombocytopenia.

PORTABLE CHEST AND ABDOMEN: Comparison is made with the previous study of July 5, 1999. The examination of the chest is essentially unchanged.

Examination of the abdomen is compared with the previous study of July 5, 1999. Interval placement of a right femoral central venous catheter with the tip within the proximal right common iliac vein near the bifurcation, at the level of the L3 vertebral body.[1]The rest of the examination is otherwise unchanged. Again, intraluminal contrast is seen within the cecum and right colon.

IMPRESSION

1. Status post placement of right common iliac central venous catheter.
2. Otherwise unchanged examination of the chest and abdomen.

Footnotes:

1. 1.Read this sentence out loud...it is not a complete sentence. Dictators frequently do this. Often it is preferred to edit the information as dictated—incomplete sentences and all.

CLINICAL HISTORY: An 83-year-old African-American male status post Hickman placement.

PORTABLE CHEST: A right central venous catheter is seen via subclavian venous approach with the tip within the superior vena cava. Diffuse patchy infiltrates with perihilar[1]predominance are seen bilaterally. This may represent adult respiratory distress syndrome versus lymphatic spread of tumor. Superimposed fluid overload may also exist in either case. The heart size, however, appears normal, and the overall aeration is not markedly diminished. No evidence of pleural effusions or pneumothoraces.

IMPRESSION: Diffuse patchy infiltrates with perihilar predominance. In the absence of old films this probably represents lymphangitic spread of tumor with superimposed fluid overload. If the patient has received chemotherapy in the recent past, this may also represent a post chemotherapeutic autoimmune response. Clinical correlation[2] is advised.

Footnotes:

1. 1.Peri means around and hilar refers to the hilum, so perihilar means around the hilum.
2. 2.Clinical correlation is a common phrase in radiology (and other medical specialties). It means to verify current findings through additional types of examination.

SPELLING.
Determine if the following words are spelled correctly. If the spelling is correct, leave the word as it has already been entered. If the spelling is incorrect, provide the correct spelling.

1. sublcavian _____

2. gleniod fossa _____

3. proximle _____

4. periphral _____

5. cephalic _____

MATCHING.
Match the correct term to the definition.

1. ____ Pertaining to inflammation of a lymphatic vessel. A. pneumothorax

2. ____ Of or relating to the hipbone. B. lymphangitic

3. ____ Abnormally low number of platelets in the blood. C. superimposed

4. ____ Placed on or over something. D. thrombocytopenia

5. ____ Abnormal presence of air in the chest outside the lung. E. iliac

ULTRASOUND REPORTS 1–3

CLINICAL HISTORY: Microhematuria.[1]

BILATERAL RENAL ULTRASOUND: The right kidney measures approximately 12.6 cm in longitudinal diameter by 4.6 cm in AP dimension by 5.8 cm in mediolateral dimension. Right collecting system measures approximately 2 x 3.3 cm in AP and mediolateral dimensions respectively and is compatible with an extrarenal pelvis. No caliectasis[2] is seen. Renal echogenicity is otherwise normal on the right. The left kidney measures approximately 13.7 cm in superoinferior dimension by 6 cm in AP dimension by 5.9 cm in mediolateral dimension. A small 8-mm echogenic focus is noted in the left upper pole compatible with calculus. No hydronephrosis is seen, and renal echogenicity is otherwise normal. No extrarenal pelvis[3] is seen on the left.

IMPRESSION

1. Prominent right extrarenal pelvis.
2. An 8-mm left upper pole calculus. Otherwise normal left kidney.

Footnotes:

1. 1. If you aren't sure what this word means, break it down (or look it up).
2. 2. Caliectasis means dilation of the calices and is often a result of obstruction or infection. This term can be used interchangeably with calicectasis.
3. 3. The renal pelvis is an expansion of the upper end of the ureter; when a portion of this expansion is located outside the kidney it is called an extrarenal pelvis.

CLINICAL HISTORY: 62-year-old female status post CABG[1] times 5, respiratory arrest, with what appears to be an effusion. Would appreciate ultrasound to determine extent of fluid.

ULTRASOUND, LEFT THORAX: Real-time ultrasound was performed on the left hemithorax. Below the diaphragm, a normal left kidney was identified measuring approximately 9 x 5 x 4.5 cm. The spleen was seen and appeared normal. Within the left thorax, a large subpulmonic effusion is identified, whose maximal dimensions measure approximately 7 cm in superior/inferior dimension by 8 cm in anteroposterior dimension.

IMPRESSION: Large left subpulmonic effusion.

Footnotes:

1. 1.This is pronounced cabbage and stands for coronary artery bypass grafting.

CLINICAL HISTORY: A 52-year-old Caucasian male status post colon resection for CA in 1996, with biopsy of undifferentiated squamous cell carcinoma with increased AST, ALT. Please evaluate. Rule out liver mets.

The liver appears within normal parameters. However, the gallbladder appears contracted at 1400 hours despite a history of no oral intake since breakfast. There is a suggestion of some debris versus stones within the gallbladder. There is no evidence of biliary duct dilatation. Images of the spleen, kidneys, and region of the pancreas appear unremarkable. However, there is a question of a generous sized right adrenal, which appears full, measuring approximately 3.2 cm in length, with an AP dimension of 1.7 cm.

IMPRESSION

1. Contracted gallbladder with possible gallstones versus debris. Recommend repeat exam after the patient has been fasting overnight.
2. Query right adrenal mass. Recommend CT to exclude adrenal pathology.

SPELLING.

Determine if the following words are spelled correctly. If the spelling is correct, leave the word as it has already been entered. If the spelling is incorrect, provide the correct spelling.

1. calliectasis _____

2. subpulmonic _____

3. anterioposterior _____

4. hemithorax _____

5. efusion _____

Multiple Choice.

Choose the best answer.

1. Ultrasound revealed no evidence of (⬭ billiary, ⬭ biliary) duct dilatation.

2. No (⬭ hydronephrosis, ⬭ hydronaphrosis) is seen.

3. The (⬭ splean, ⬭ spleen) appeared normal.

4. Renal (⬭ echogenicity, ⬭ echogenacity) is normal on the right.

5. There is a suggestion of some debris (⬭ verses, ⬭ versus) stones within the gallbladder.

ULTRASOUND REPORT 4

CLINICAL HISTORY: Confirm dates.

OBSTETRICAL ULTRASOUND

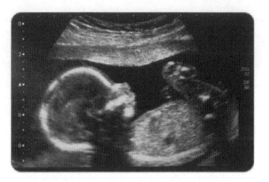

BPD[1] is 5.1 cm (age by ultrasound is 21.3 weeks). Occipitofrontal diameter is 6.9 cm, and head circumference is 19.1 cm (age by ultrasound is 21.4 weeks). Abdominal diameter is 5.6 cm, and abdominal circumference is 17.5 cm (age by ultrasound 22.4 weeks). Femur length is 3.6 cm (age by ultrasound 21.4 weeks). Average age by ultrasound is 21.3 weeks. Age by dates have an LMP of December 10, 2005, which is 20.3 weeks. Estimated fetal weight is 484 gm. Head circumference/abdominal circumference ratio is 1:10.

On review of anatomy, intracranial contents appear unremarkable without evidence of ventriculomegaly.[2] Spine is followed as well as the sacrum. A 4-chamber view of the heart is obtained. The fetal stomach, kidneys, and bladder are identified. Umbilical cord insertion appears intact with a 3-vessel cord.

IMPRESSION

1. Minimal discrepancy between size and dates with EDC as calculated by ultrasound. Ultrasonic dating should be accurate +/-10[3] days at this stage of gestation.
2. Fibroid uterus.

Footnotes:

1. 1. BPD = biparietal diameter is the diameter of fetal head from one parietal eminence to the other. BPD is one of a variety of measurements taken to gauge gestational age.
2. 2. Breaking it down, we know that ventriculomegaly means abnormally large ventricle of the brain (which can occur in hydrocephalus).
3. 3. This could be acceptably edited as plus minus 10 days.

SPELLING.
Determine if the following words are spelled correctly. If the spelling is correct, leave the word as it has already been entered. If the spelling is incorrect, provide the correct spelling.

1. ventriculomegaly _____

2. femer _____

3. occipitofrontal _____

4. circumfrence _____

5. intrauterine _____

FILL IN THE BLANK.
Using the word(s) in the box, enter the appropriate term in the space provided.

1. The patient's last _____ period was in December.

2. Ultrasound revealed no evidence of placenta _____.

3. The amount of _____ fluid is normal.

4. No enlarged ventricles are seen on review of _____ contents.

5. Exam reveals a 3-vessel _____.

| amniotic |
| cord |
| intracranial |
| menstrual |
| previa |

ULTRASOUND REPORT 5

CLINICAL HISTORY: Left CVA[1] with left carotid stenosis/occlusion. Please assess for flow.

CAROTID DOPPLER STUDY

On the right side there is arteriosclerotic plaque noted at the level of the carotid bulb along the ventral aspect with acoustic shadowing. This plaque measures approximately 7–8 mm in length. It is difficult to assess the AP dimension due to the shadowing. There is some plaque also noted at the origin of the internal carotid artery, which appears predominantly fibrinous, measuring approximately 8 mm in length along the ventral wall with an AP dimension of approximately 3 mm. It is more difficult to evaluate the dorsal wall. On Doppler spectral analysis, the peak systolic velocity in the common carotid artery is 0.62 meters per second[2] and in the internal carotid artery margin at its greatest 0.91 meters per second for a ratio of approximately 1.5. The flow more distally in the internal carotid artery is slightly lower with a peak velocity of 0.78 meters per second in the mid internal carotid artery, and 0.83 meters per second distally. Antegrade flow was documented within the right vertebral artery.

On the left side, there is intimal thickening noted in the common carotid artery, with extensive plaque in the level of the bulb extending into the origin of the internal carotid artery. The plaque appears all fibrinous, with almost total or total occlusion of the proximal internal carotid artery. On Doppler spectral analysis, the flow appears dampened in the common carotid artery as compared to the right, with peak systolic velocity of 0.45 meters per second. At the level of the margin, there is almost a stump phenomenon. However, on careful Doppler spectral analysis, a jet was identified with a peak systolic velocity greater than 4 meters per second with an end diastolic velocity of approximately 3 meters per second. There was turbulence throughout the cardiac cycle. Antegrade flow was documented within the left external carotid artery and right external carotid artery, as well as antegrade flow in the vertebral artery.

IMPRESSION: Approximately 50% stenosis of the right internal carotid artery with extremely tight, approximately 99%, stenosis of the proximal left internal carotid artery.

Footnotes:

1. 1.CVA = cerebrovascular accident. (Note, CVA also stands for costovertebral angle tenderness, but since this is a carotid Doppler study, you can be sure the correct expansion is cerebrovascular accident.)
2. 2.Meters per second can also be edited as m/s or m/sec.

SPELLING.
Determine if the following words are spelled correctly. If the spelling is correct, leave the word as it has already been entered. If the spelling is incorrect, provide the correct spelling.

1. caratid _____

2. fibrinus _____

3. oclusion _____

4. systolic _____

5. cerebrovasculer _____

MATCHING.

Match the correct term to the definition.

1. ____ Situated nearest the point of origin.

2. ____ Relating to the innermost membrane of an organ.

3. ____ Hardened arterial walls.

4. ____ An abnormal narrowing of a passageway.

5. ____ In the direction of normal movement.

A. stenosis

B. intimal

C. antegrade

D. arteriosclerotic

E. proximal

MRI REPORTS 1–2

CLINICAL HISTORY: Episodes of cortical blindness, vertigo, nausea, and headache. Possible vertebral basilar TIAs.[1]

MRI OF THE BRAIN

PROCEDURE: Sagittal and axial T1 weighted images were obtained through the brain, followed by proton density and T2 weighted images in the axial plane. Finally, post-Magnevist administration axial images were obtained with T1 weighting.

FINDINGS: The ventricles are of normal size, shape, and configuration. No abnormal areas of increased T2 weighted signal or post-contrast areas of increased signal are appreciated. No evidence of infarct. There are no abnormal intra- or extra-axial fluid collections identified. Specifically, the cortical regions and posterior fossa are within normal limits. The basilar artery shows normal signal void.

IMPRESSION

1. Normal MRI of the brain, including post-Magnevist injection images.[2]

Footnotes:

1. 1.TIA = transient ischemic attack is a brief episode or attack where there is not enough blood supplied to the brain.
2. 2.Again, generally you would not list a #1 without at least a #2. This MTE did edit a 1 without a 2, and without specific instruction regarding lists, this is acceptable.

CLINICAL HISTORY: A 49-year-old female with DJD at C5-6 and right neural foraminal narrowing on plain films.

PROCEDURE: Sagittal T1 and MPGR images were obtained through the cervical spine, followed by MPGR images in the axial plane through the cervical spine.

FINDINGS: There is spinal stenosis at the C4-5 and C5-6 levels, caused by a congenitally narrow anterior/posterior diameter of the spinal canal with superimposed posterior vertebral osteophytes at these levels. In addition, there is a small right paracentral/lateral focal disk protrusion at the C4-5 level. There is also hypertrophy of the facets at the C5-6 level, which results in moderate neural foraminal narrowing bilaterally at this level.

IMPRESSION

1. Spinal stenosis at C4-5 and C5-6 levels, caused by congenitally narrow spinal canal with posterior vertebral osteophytes at this level.
2. Focal right paracentral disk protrusion at C4-5 level, with probable impingement on right C5 nerve root.
3. Bilateral neural foraminal narrowing at C5-6 level.

SPELLING.
Determine if the following words are spelled correctly. If the spelling is correct, leave the word as it has already been entered. If the spelling is incorrect, provide the correct spelling.

1. facet _____

2. foramanal _____

3. Magnevist _____

4. paricentral _____

5. basillar _____

MULTIPLE CHOICE.

Choose the correct spelling of the term.

1. A spinning or whirling sensation.

   ○ vertago

   ○ vertego

   ○ vertigo

   ○ virtigo

2. A bony outgrowth.

   ○ osteophyte

   ○ ostiophyte

   ○ osteophyt

   ○ osteophite

3. A two-dimensional flat surface.

   ○ plain

   ○ plaine

   ○ playne

   ○ plane

4. MPGR

   ○ multiplanar graded recalled

   ○ multiplanar gradient recall

   ○ multiplanner gradient recalc

   ○ multiplaner graded recall

5. Abnormal enlargement of an organ.

   ○ hypotrophy

   ○ hypertrophy

   ○ hypatrophy

   ○ hypertraphy

MRI REPORTS 3–4

MRI OF THE BRAIN

PROCEDURE: Axial and sagittal T1 weighted images were obtained through the brain, followed by proton density and T2 weighted images in the axial plane.

FINDINGS: There is extensive, diffuse cerebral atrophy, manifest by increased size of the ventricles and cortical sulci. In addition, there is focal loss of cortex in the right frontoparietal and parietooccipital regions, where there are also extensive areas of increased proton density and T2 weighted signal involving both the white matter and gray matter. These are consistent with old right frontoparietal and right parietooccipital infarcts. In addition, there are multiple small foci of increased proton density and T2 weighted signal in the periventricular and centrum semiovale white matter, consistent with small vessel ischemic change. Furthermore, there are focal areas of increased proton density and T2 weighted signal in the left basal ganglia, consistent with small lacunar infarctions. Incidentally noted is increased signal in the ethmoid air cells, consistent with sinusitis. Maxillary, sphenoid, and frontal sinuses are clear.

IMPRESSION

1. Old right frontoparietal and parietooccipital infarcts.
2. Old lacunar infarcts of left basal ganglia.
3. Small vessel ischemic changes.
4. Diffuse cerebral atrophy.
5. Ethmoid sinusitis.

CLINICAL HISTORY: A 24-year-old male complaining of pain on palpation of upper T-spine, with abnormal curvature of C-spine on plain film. CT scan recommended by radiology.

MRI OF THE CERVICAL SPINE: T1 sagittal, fast spin echo, variable echo sagittal, and MPGR axial images of the cervical spine were obtained.

C2-3, C3-4, C4-5, C7-T1[1] are without abnormality. Both nerve roots are without impingement. There is no evidence of disk bulge or impingement upon the thecal sac.

C5-6 demonstrates central and left paracentral HNP with impression upon the thecal sac without direct impingement upon the nerve roots.

C6-7 demonstrates central HNP with impression upon the thecal sac. There is no impingement upon the nerve roots bilaterally.

IMPRESSION

1. C5-6 central and left paracentral HNP without impingement upon the nerve roots.
2. C6-7 central herniated nucleus pulposus without impingement upon the nerve roots.
3. The remainder of the cervical spine is without abnormality.

Footnotes:

1. 1.Per the *BOS*, it is not necessary to repeat the same letter before the second vertebra when listing intervertebral disk spaces, but it may be edited when dictated (C1-2 and/or C1-C2).

SPELLING.
Determine if the following words are spelled correctly. If the spelling is correct, leave the word as it has already been entered. If the spelling is incorrect, provide the correct spelling.

1. sagital _____

2. centrum semivale _____

3. ishcemic _____

4. pulposus _____

5. atraphy _____

TRUE/FALSE.

Mark the following true or false.

1. In the brain MRI, the maxillary, sphenoid, ethmoid, and frontal sinuses are clear.

    ○ true

    ○ false

2. Fast spin echo views were taken in the cervical spine MRI.

    ○ true

    ○ false

3. Spine MRI shows no nerve root impingement.

    ○ true

    ○ false

4. HNP, as used in the cervical spine MRI, stands for herniated nucleus pulposus.

    ○ true

    ○ false

5. The MRI of the brain is performed with no significant findings.

    ○ true

    ○ false

CT SCAN REPORTS 1–2

CLINICAL HISTORY: Status post excision of lesion of skull. Postop MRI showed a clival lesion.[1]

CT OF THE BRAIN

PROCEDURE: Sagittal T1 weighted images were obtained through the region of the clivus both pre- and post-Magnevist injection.

FINDINGS: The pre-Magnevist injection images demonstrate some replacement of the normal marrow fat expected in the clivus. However, these images do not demonstrate any focal lesion. However, on the post-Magnevist injection there is a 3–4 mm low signal lesion with faint peripheral enhancement. These findings are consistent with eosinophilic granuloma of the clivus. There is no evidence of cortical disruption or bony expansion. The sphenoid sinus is clear. Limited views of the maxillary sinuses and ethmoid sinuses are unremarkable. The visualized portions of the brain are unremarkable.

IMPRESSION: Findings compatible with eosinophilic granuloma of clivus. However, no evidence of cortical disruption or bony expansion.

Footnotes:

1. 1.A clival lesion is one pertaining to the clivus. (If you aren't completely sure where the clivus is you can probably figure out the general area by the content, but it would be a good idea to look it up to be sure.)

CLINICAL HISTORY: Myoclonic jerks. Rule out focal lesion. BB in face, and therefore cannot do MRI.

CT SCAN OF THE HEAD: 10 x 10 mm contiguous cuts through the brain without contrast with additional 5 x 5 mm contiguous cuts through the posterior fossa and continued 5 x 7 mm cuts through the remainder of the head with contrast.

No mass, midline shift, or bleed is noted. The ventricles and sulci are within normal limits. No vascular abnormalities are seen. The bones are within normal limits. What is seen of the orbits and sinuses is without abnormality.

IMPRESSION: Normal head.

SPELLING.
Determine if the following words are spelled correctly. If the spelling is correct, leave the word as it has already been entered. If the spelling is incorrect, provide the correct spelling.

1. cortical _____

2. sulci _____

3. fosa _____

4. clivous _____

5. contigous _____

MATCHING.
Match the correct term to the definition.

1. ____ A displacement of the midline of the brain to one side of the head due to swelling.

2. ____ Disease marked by formation of granulomas in the bone.

3. ____ Relating to an external layer.

4. ____ Difference in visual density in an x-ray that results from a difference in radiolucency of the subject.

5. ____ A contraction or spasm of a portion of a muscle, a whole muscle, or a group of muscles.

A. myoclonic

B. eosinophilic granuloma

C. midline shift

D. contrast

E. cortical

CT SCAN REPORTS 3–4

CLINICAL HISTORY: Status post choledochojejunostomy, gastrojejunostomy, and small bowel follow through which suggests sinus tract. Please evaluate.

CT SCAN OF THE ABDOMEN

PROCEDURE: Contiguous[1] 5 mm sections were obtained through the upper abdomen without the administration of intravenous contrast, although oral contrast was administered on a prior Gastrografin upper GI series.

There is a linear collection of high density just medial to the anastomotic suture line which projects in the right upper quadrant. This corresponds to the area of linear high density on the Gastrografin upper GI series and is suggestive of a sinus tract. Surgical clips are seen in the region of the gallbladder fossa, and there is linear high attenuation noted in the region of the gastrohepatic ligament, suggestive of reflux into the biliary tree from choledochojejunostomy.

IMPRESSION

1. Findings compatible with sinus tract filled with contrast from Gastrografin upper gastrointestinal series.
2. No evidence of abscess or mass.

Footnotes:

1. 1.Contiguous means touching or connected throughout in an unbroken sequence.

CLINICAL HISTORY: A 67-year-old female with complaints consistent with spinal stenosis, status post L2-S1 laminectomy.

LUMBAR MYELOGRAM: The patient was advised as to the risks and benefits of the procedure and gave her informed consent in writing. The skin over the L2-3 area was prepped and draped in a sterile fashion and anesthetized with 1% Xylocaine. A 22 gauge spinal needle was inserted into the spinal canal and position was verified using fluoro.[1] Then 2 cc of Omnipaque 240 contrast was[2] injected into the spinal canal, and myelographic images, as well as CT images, were obtained of the lumbar spine. On the lateral myelographic image, there were disk bulges at L1-2, L3-4, and L4-5. CT images demonstrate a right paracentral HNP at L1-2, together with facet hypertrophy, and ligamentum flavum hypertrophy produces moderate spinal stenosis. At L2-3 there is evidence of prior laminectomy, and there remains facet hypertrophy and ligamentum flavum hypertrophy, producing moderate canal stenosis. At L3-4 there is evidence of prior laminectomy. There remains facet hypertrophy, which produces moderate spinal canal stenosis. At L4-5 there is facet hypertrophy and evidence of prior laminectomy. At L5-S1 there is facet hypertrophy, which produces significant spinal stenosis.

IMPRESSION

1. Multilevel degenerative changes of the lumbar spine with moderately severe spinal stenosis at the L1-2 level, produced by a left paracentral HNP, together with facet hypertrophy and ligamentum flavum hypertrophy.
2. Moderate spinal stenosis at L2-3, L3-4, and L4-5 produced by facet hypertrophy. The patient appears to be status post laminectomy of L2-S1.

Footnotes:

1. 1.Fluoro is slang or short for fluoroscopy.
2. 2.Even if dictated "were," the correct tense is "was." Units of measurement are treated as a collective singular noun (2 cc *was*, not 2 cc *were* injected).

SPELLING.
Determine if the following words are spelled correctly. If the spelling is correct, leave the word as it has already been entered. If the spelling is incorrect, provide the correct spelling.

1. Gastrograffin _____
2. hypertrophy _____
3. abcess _____
4. Omnipaque _____
5. choledochojejunestomy _____

MULTIPLE CHOICE.
Choose the best answer.

1. Abdominal CT findings are suggestive of a sinus (○ tract, ○ track).
2. CT was performed in (○ continuous, ○ contiguous) 5 mm sections.
3. Lumbar myelogram reveals there is still ligamentum (○ flavim, ○ flavum) hypertrophy.
4. Patient is status post (○ lamenectomy, ○ laminectomy) of L2-S1.
5. CT scan of the abdomen is suggestive of (○ reflux, ○ reflex) into the biliary tree.

CONTRAST STUDY REPORTS 1–2

CLINICAL HISTORY: 59-year-old with history of melena, evaluated by endoscopy, which revealed small duodenal erosions and nonsteroidal anti-inflammatory drug[1] gastritis. Colonic AVMs were felt to be the source of bleeding. Patient now with iron-deficiency anemia.

SMALL BOWEL ENTEROCLYSIS:[2]After placement of a catheter, barium was instilled followed by 0.5% methylcellulose. Several 0.7-mm round filling defects were identified in the distal ileum on multiple views. These are felt to represent air bubbles or food material. However, small polyps cannot be entirely excluded. No other small intestinal abnormalities were identified.

IMPRESSION

1. Multiple small filling defects within the distal ileum that most likely represent air bubbles or food material. However, small polyps cannot be excluded.
2. Otherwise, normal small bowel.

Footnotes:

1. 1.Nonsteroidal anti-inflammatory (also acceptably edited as antiinflammatory) drugs are commonly referred to as NSAIDs.
2. 2.This report was edited with the term "enterocleisis." The term *enterocleisis* refers to a blockage in the alimentary canal. However, enteroclysis is a radiographic procedure. Here is where soundalikes and verifying content come into play! Always make sure what you hear makes sense!

CLINICAL HISTORY: A 60-year-old with CREST.[1]

CINE ESOPHAGRAM:[2] The patient ingested a barium meal without any difficulties. There is evidence of mitral valve replacement. Small calcific densities are seen in the splenic area. There is mild right lower lobe fibrosis. On the esophagram there is no significant esophageal motility. No evidence of gastroesophageal reflux. No evidence of dilation of the esophagus. Review of the cine esophagram showed normal progression of barium meal throughout all segments of the esophagus. No evidence of cricopharyngeal abnormality demonstrated.

IMPRESSION

1. Normal cine esophagram.
2. Normal esophageal motility.

Footnotes:

1. 1.CREST stands for calcinosis cutis, Raynaud phenomenon, esophageal motility disorder, sclerodactyly, and telangiectasia syndrome.
2. 2.Cine is pronounced seenay.

SPELLING.
Determine if the following words are spelled correctly. If the spelling is correct, leave the word as it has already been entered. If the spelling is incorrect, provide the correct spelling.

1. calcific _____   2. cricopharyingeal _____

3. esophagis _____   4. melana _____

5. enteroclysis _____

MULTIPLE CHOICE.
Choose the best answer.

1. AVM stands for (○ atriovenous, ○ arteriovenous) malformation.
2. The patient (○ engested, ○ ingested) barium without any difficulties.
3. NSAID stands for (○ nonstroidal, ○ nonsteroidal) anti-inflammatory drug
4. Small (○ polyps, ○ polyaps) cannot be excluded.
5. There is no evidence of (○ gastroesophageal, ○ gastroeosophageal) reflux.

CONTRAST STUDY REPORTS 3–4

CLINICAL HISTORY: Right abdominal pain, rule out diverticulitis.

BARIUM ENEMA: The barium flowed freely from the rectum to the cecum. However, the colon is extremely redundant, particularly for this age patient, and initially it was difficult to obtain coating of the cecum and ascending colon. There is a moderate amount of retained fecal material. However, the colon otherwise appears unremarkable without evidence of spasm, persistent narrowing, mass, or mass effect. No diverticula are identified.

IMPRESSION: Large caliber redundant colon, within normal variation. Exam otherwise unremarkable.

CLINICAL HISTORY: A 6-day-old infant with right UPJ obstruction. Needs lower tract evaluation.

VOIDING CYSTOURETHROGRAM: 75 cc of Urovist is allowed to flow into the bladder via a catheter. The bladder shape is normal. There is no reflux demonstrated. Voiding is initiated spontaneously. Approximately 10 cc of urine remains in the bladder following completion of voiding.

IMPRESSION

1. No reflux of contrast into the ureters.
2. No other abnormalities seen.

SPELLING.
Determine if the following words are spelled correctly. If the spelling is correct, leave the word as it has already been entered. If the spelling is incorrect, provide the correct spelling.

1. spontanously _____

2. Uravist _____

3. obstruction _____

4. redundant _____

5. asending _____

MATCHING.
Match the correct term to the definition.

1. ____ Junction of the renal pelvis and the ureter.

2. ____ The pouch in which the large intestine begins.

3. ____ Herniation through the muscular wall of a tubular organ that has become inflamed.

4. ____ An abnormally backward flow of body fluids.

5. ____ Discharging waste matter, usually referencing urination.

A. diverticulitis

B. ureteropelvic junction

C. cecum

D. voiding

E. reflux

CONTRAST STUDY REPORT 5

CLINICAL HISTORY: The patient is 13 days postoperative from exploratory celiotomy for pancreatic mass. Palliative diverting procedure was performed at the same time. The patient progressed well with Gastrografin study last week showing patent anastomosis and stomach emptying. The patient started slowly on liquids without complaints until yesterday when the patient complained of abdominal pain, emesis x1, and no bowel movement. Bowel sounds persistently absent. Please check anastomosis and stomach emptying.

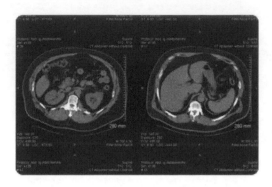

On plain films of the upper abdomen, there are multiple surgical clips and staples. Surgical clips are noted at the level of the GE junction, consistent with a history of vagotomy. There are surgical clips at the level of the gallbladder fossa just to the left of L1, consistent with gastrojejunal anastomosis. There are also surgical staples noted just to the right of L2-3, at approximately the level of the choledochojejunostomy. This was not evaluated in detail. The patient slowly sipped Gastrografin. The residual stomach appears unremarkable with no evidence of anastomotic leak at the gastrojejunostomy. There is good filling of the efferent loop with a suggestion of only minimal bowel wall thickening of the proximal efferent loop. There is some filling of the afferent loop, approximately 6 cm. At the most proximal aspect of the demonstrated afferent loop, there is some puddling of contrast, which most likely is contrast within the biliary tree with individual small areas of contrast measuring approximately 3 mm, although there is lack of good demonstration of the intrahepatic biliary system.

[1] There is also a slightly irregular linear density of contrast which extends caudal and to the right of the afferent loop, measuring approximately 7 cm in length with a width as great as 1–2 mm. It is uncertain within what structure this linear collection of contrast is. It is conceivable it is part of the afferent loop, but a fistulous tract cannot be excluded. It is at approximately a 90-degree angle to the probable axis of the common bile duct, and if this represents pancreatic duct it is filling in a direction of the midbody to the head of the pancreas.

On delayed 1-hour film there is contrast noted all the way to the level of below the rectum. The previously described linear collection of contrast to the right of the afferent loop is again identified, unchanged in appearance, but meanwhile there has been further emptying of the afferent loop.

IMPRESSION

1. Inversion procedure, as described above, with good filling of the efferent loop without evidence of obstruction.
2. Possible fistulous tract or unusual appearance of afferent loop. This case has been discussed with Dr. Mornay and Dr. Stevens, and it may be of benefit to obtain thin section CT scan through the right upper quadrant for further assessment of the contrast collection.

Footnotes:

1. 1. This is a pretty long run-on sentence. If account instructions allow for minor editing, it might be okay to break it up a bit.

SPELLING.
Determine if the following words are spelled correctly. If the spelling is correct, leave the word as it has already been entered. If the spelling is incorrect, provide the correct spelling.

1. obstuction _____

2. aferent _____

3. gastrojejunel _____

4. inversion _____

5. pancraetic _____

FILL IN THE BLANK.

Using the word(s) in the box, enter the appropriate term in the space provided.

1. An _____ loop is directed away from the center.

2. A _____ is an abdominal incision.

3. A surgical _____ is the joining of parts or branches to become continuous.

4. An abnormal passage between two organs or from an organ to the body surface.

    _____

5. Treatment performed to reduce severity of symptoms or disease. _____

anastomosis
celiotomy
efferent
fistula
palliative

MAMMOGRAPHY REPORT 1

CLINICAL HISTORY: Annual followup.

BILATERAL MAMMOGRAM: Comparison is made with the prior study from June 2005. Since the prior exam there has been interim development of a soft tissue density of a somewhat ovoid shape at approximately the 9:30 position in the left breast, adjacent to the thoracic wall. This demonstrates somewhat ill-defined margins. However, no definite spiculations,[1] architectural distortion, or clustered microcalcifications are seen within it. Maximum dimensions are about 1 cm. The region of palpable concern in the left upper outer quadrant is grossly unremarkable on mammographic study. The right breast is not significantly changed, and no suspicious findings are seen.

Ultrasound was performed on this date on the left breast, which did not confirm cyst in the medial portion of the breast, for the lesion described above.

IMPRESSION: New soft tissue density in the medial left breast, as described above. This cannot be confirmed as a simple cyst. Therefore, needle localization biopsy was recommended to the patient. The patient accepted this offer and is scheduled for biopsy on June 2, 2006. The case was discussed with Dr. Clark.

Footnotes:

1. 1.A spicule is a small needle-shaped body.

SPELLING.
Determine if the following words are spelled correctly. If the spelling is correct, leave the word as it has already been entered. If the spelling is incorrect, provide the correct spelling.

1. microcalcifecations _____

2. quadarant _____

3. suspicious _____

4. cyst _____

5. localazation _____

MULTIPLE CHOICE.

Choose the correct spelling of the term.

1. Rounded like an egg.

   ○ oviod

   ○ ovioid

   ○ ovoid

   ○ ovioud

2. Quality of being compact.

   ○ dense

   ○ dens

   ○ dinse

   ○ denise

3. Of or relating to the chest.

   ○ thracic

   ○ thoracic

   ○ thoracec

   ○ thorocic

4. The state of being out of normal shape or position.

   ○ distrortion

   ○ distorshun

   ○ dictortion

   ○ distortion

5. A pathologic change in the tissue.

   ○ leshun

   ○ lesoin

   ○ lesion

   ○ lesione

MAMMOGRAPHY REPORTS 2–3

CLINICAL HISTORY: The patient had a left mastectomy in the fall of 1996 for infiltrating ductal carcinoma. No current problems with the right breast.

RIGHT MAMMOGRAM: The right breast is radiographically unchanged compared to the March 2007[1] study and continues to show no evidence of malignancy.

IMPRESSION

1. Radiographically stable breast without evidence of malignancy.
2. The patient has been advised to continue annual radiographic screening.

Footnotes:

1. 1. You do not need a comma after the year when the day is not dictated.

CLINICAL HISTORY: Baseline.

BILATERAL MAMMOGRAM: Exam is a baseline exam. The breasts are somewhat radiodense bilaterally. In the upper outer quadrant of the left breast, approximately the 2 o'clock position,[1] there is a small cluster of calcifications. These calcifications are less than 0.5 mm, and there are approximately 8 within a cubic cm. Morphology is slightly irregular; however, definite linear morphology is not appreciated. No definite architectural distortion or associated soft tissue mass is seen within the region. The remainder of the breasts are free of suspicious findings.

IMPRESSION: Clustered microcalcifications in the left upper outer quadrant, as described above. Findings were felt to be suspicious enough to recommend needle localization and biopsy of this region. The patient was counseled regarding these findings and agreed to needle localization and biopsy, which had been scheduled on January 28, 2007, at 9 a.m. in the mammography department.

Footnotes:

1. 1.When editing positions it is generally preferred to use "o'clock" instead of :00. This wouldn't be feasible, of course, for those half-hour notations.

SPELLING.
Determine if the following words are spelled correctly. If the spelling is correct, leave the word as it has already been entered. If the spelling is incorrect, provide the correct spelling.

1. quadrent _____

2. counsled _____

3. baseline _____

4. radiodense _____

5. mastectimy _____

MULTIPLE CHOICE.
Choose the best answer.

1. The patient had a mastectomy for (○ infaltrating, ○ infiltrating) ductal carcinoma.
2. Right mammogram shows no evidence of (○ malignancy, ○ malignency).
3. The patient's (○ morphalogy, ○ morphology) is slightly irregular.
4. The breasts are free of (○ suspicious, ○ suspicous) findings.
5. There is no definite (○ agricultural, ○ architectural) distortion seen.

THERAPEUTIC RADIOLOGY REPORTS

Therapeutic radiology involves the use of radiation for treatment of disease. This is a very broad definition, and there are a variety of subcategories that fall under the umbrella of therapeutic radiology.

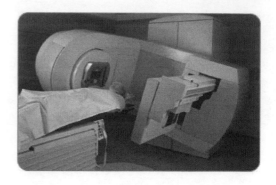

Radiation Therapy– The use of radiation for treatment of disease.

Interventional Radiology– The use of image guidance for therapeutic and angiographic procedures.

Nuclear Medicine– The use of radioactive materials to identify or destroy lesions and disease processes.

Radiation therapy is the subcategory we will be focusing on in this portion of the radiology unit. Radiation therapy is a treatment for cancer. Radiation can be used to cure cancer or to alleviate a cancer patient's pain. It is usually done in conjunction with chemotherapy, and can be done on most parts of the body. The types of reports encountered in radiation therapy are consultation reports, which are basically detailed histories and physical examinations to determine the need for radiation therapy; procedure reports, which include dates and times, fields, and dosage of radiation; and finally progress notes, or followup examinations of patients after they have completed their course of radiation therapy.

The following are just a small sampling of radiation therapy reports.

THERAPEUTIC RADIOLOGY REPORT 1

PATIENT PROFILE: A 59-year-old male with medullary carcinoma of the thyroid.

HISTORY: Mr. Mitchell first noted a right neck mass in January and presented to the hospital at that time. He was evaluated extensively and ultimately underwent a total thyroidectomy in early February. Final pathology of the thyroidectomy revealed medullary carcinoma of the thyroid in both lobes, as well as 3 adjacent lymph nodes positive for metastatic disease. He was subsequently referred to Oncology where his postoperative calcitonin level[1] was recorded at 8960. Further evaluation with MRI to the neck revealed residual disease in the neck, and he underwent a right modified radical neck dissection in April, revealing 19 of 40 lymph nodes involved with metastatic disease. He has recovered nicely from the surgery, having had a parathyroid transplant to preserve his parathyroid function. He states that he is feeling well, has maintained a stable weight, and has noted no lumps or bumps and no hoarseness.

PHYSICAL EXAMINATION: None performed.

DIAGNOSTIC STUDIES: CT of the chest reports no evidence of metastatic disease and no extension of the right neck mass into the chest. MRI scan of the neck reports a nodular soft tissue density, measuring 2 x 1 cm, to the right of the trachea and the esophagus at the level of the sternal notch, which could represent either a lymph node or residual thyroid tissue. Final pathology from the right modified neck dissection reports a benign scar, benign thymic tissue, and 19 out of 40 lymph nodes positive for metastatic medullary carcinoma of the thyroid. Of note, there is no pericapsular extension, and the margins of resection are negative.

IMPRESSION

1. Locally advanced medullary carcinoma of the thyroid, status post total thyroidectomy and subsequent right modified radical neck dissection with 19 of 40 nodes involved with metastatic disease, without extracapsular extension and with negative surgical margins.
2. Unknown extended disease in the left neck.

RECOMMENDATIONS

1. I agree with the plan to dissect the left neck to further evaluate for metastatic disease in the left neck nodes.
2. I would recommend a postoperative calcitonin level following the left neck dissection as an indicator for residual disease.
3. This patient may warrant a full evaluation by Endocrinology to rule out MEN syndromes[2] if not already performed.
4. If there is any evidence for residual disease in the neck, the patient may be a candidate for postoperative adjuvant radiation therapy. Please reconsult after his surgery and calcitonin level have been completed.

Footnotes:

1. 1.Calcitonin levels greater than 100 pg/mL may occur in medullary thyroid carcinoma (MTC), leukemia, and myeloproliferative disorders.
2. 2.MEN = multiple endocrine neoplasia. MEN syndromes are conditions that result in overactivity and enlargement in certain endocrine glands. MEN syndromes are typically inherited conditions.

SPELLING.
Determine if the following words are spelled correctly. If the spelling is correct, leave the word as it has already been entered. If the spelling is incorrect, provide the correct spelling.

1. calctonin _____

2. extracapsular _____

3. thryoidectomy _____

4. thymic _____

5. residule _____

FILL IN THE BLANK.

Using the word(s) in the box, enter the appropriate term in the space provided.

1. When a disease spreads to another part of the body or another organ it is referred to as

   _____.

2. Cancer of the medulla of a body part is referred to as _____ carcinoma.

3. Something which is not recurrent or progressive is referred to as _____.

4. The patient had a _____ transplant.

5. A/An _____ treatment is one that is added to increase the effectiveness of

   other treatment.

adjuvant
benign
medullary
metastatic
parathyroid

THERAPEUTIC RADIOLOGY REPORT 2

PATIENT PROFILE: A 47-year-old male with pathologic stage IIIB[1] poorly differentiated adenocarcinoma of the right lung.

HISTORY: The patient first presented in December with right neck adenopathy and right hilar mass on chest x-ray. Diagnostic bronchoscopy was normal, but right supraclavicular lymph node biopsy was positive for poorly differentiated adenocarcinoma. He had some associated swelling of the right shoulder and right head consistent with early SVC syndrome.[2] He was referred for primary radiation therapy.

TREATMENT SUMMARY: The patient was treated to the lower-right neck, mediastinum, and lung using an AP/PA[3] technique with a 10 MV photon beam. This field was collimated to 18 x 23.5 cm using custom Cerrobend[4] blocking to protect normal structures. He received a daily dose of 1.8 gray 5 days a week for a total dose of 41.4 gray delivered to the 95% isodose line from February 5 through March 7, 2007.

His treatment was then changed to an off cord oblique technique with an LAO/RPO opposed pair, again using the 10 MV photon beam. This field was collimated to 14 x 23.5 cm, and again custom Cerrobend blocking was used to protect normal structures. He again received a daily dose of 1.8 gray 5 days a week for a total boost dose to the mediastinum of 19.8 gray delivered to the 93% isodose line from March 8 through March 22, 2007. This brought the total dose to the gross disease to 61.2 gray in 34 fractions over 46 elapsed days.

DISPOSITION: The patient tolerated his treatment reasonably well, experiencing some desquamation in the right supraclavicular area where 1 cm of bolus material was used to bring the superficial lymph nodes to full dose. The moist desquamation was treated conservatively with Domeboro[5] soaks with good result. He is scheduled for routine followup 4 weeks after completion of radiation therapy.

Roman numerals are typically used for cancer stages:

- stage I
- stage II
- stage III
- stage IV

Arabic numerals are typically used for cancer grades:

- grade 1
- grade 2
- grade 3
- grade 4

Footnotes:

1. 1.For subdivision of cancer stages, add capital letters or numerals on the line without spaces or hyphens (for example, stage IA, stage II3, stage IIIB).
2. 2.SVC = superior vena cava. SVC syndrome (SVCS) is a group of symptoms occurring when the superior vena cava becomes clogged or partially blocked.
3. 3.AP/PA = anteroposterior/posteroanterior positioning.
4. 4.A good radiology word book will verify the spelling of this type of block, which may be difficult to discern with complete certainty when dictated—cerabend versus serabend versus Cerrobend, etc.
5. 5.If you aren't sure what Domeboro is, look it up.

SPELLING.
Determine if the following words are spelled correctly. If the spelling is correct, leave the word as it has already been entered. If the spelling is incorrect, provide the correct spelling.

1. adenocarcinoma _____

2. hylar _____

3. colamated _____

4. desquamintion _____

5. Cerrobend _____

MULTIPLE CHOICE.

Choose the best answer.

1. SVC stands for superior (⬤ vena, ⬤ venous) cava.

2. A (⬤ Domeboro, ⬤ Domboro) soak is a therapeutic astringent solution.

3. LAO stands for left anterior (⬤ oblique, ⬤ oblicque).

4. Treatment was given using a (⬤ proton, ⬤ photon) beam.

5. MV stands for (⬤ megavolt, ⬤ millivolt).

THERAPEUTIC RADIOLOGY REPORT 3

PATIENT PROFILE: A 62-year-old male with stage IIE DHL[1] of the stomach status post 6 cycles of CHOP,[2] followed by upper abdominal radiation therapy for a total dose of 39.6 gray.

HISTORY: The patient presents today for his 2-year followup after completion of radiation therapy feeling very well. He has no B symptoms, maintains a stable weight, has noted no adenopathy, and denies other constitutional symptoms. In particular, he notes relief from his previous history of gastric cramping.

PHYSICAL EXAMINATION: General: This is a well-appearing, middle-aged male. He is alert and oriented. Lymphatics: There is no peripheral adenopathy noted. Abdomen: Soft without mass or hepatosplenomegaly.

DIAGNOSTIC STUDIES: Abdominal/pelvic CT scan reveals no evidence of tumor recurrence. Chest x-ray reveals no evidence of metastatic disease. The patient reports that a recent upper endoscopy with biopsy was normal.

IMPRESSION: No evidence of recurrent disease.

PLAN

1. The patient is to follow up for repeat examination in 3 months.
2. He is to continue to follow up with Dr. Wilson.

Footnotes:

1. 1.DHL = diffuse histiocytic lymphoma.
2. 2.CHOP is common anticancer drug combination that includes cyclophosphamide, doxorubicin, vincristine, and prednisone. Sometimes this is used in conjunction with Rituxan and may be dictated as CHOP-R (sounds like "chop R" or "chopper").

SPELLING.
Determine if the following words are spelled correctly. If the spelling is correct, leave the word as it has already been entered. If the spelling is incorrect, provide the correct spelling.

1. evidance _____

2. abdominal _____

3. hepatosplenomegaly _____

4. lymphtics _____

5. radation _____

MATCHING.

Match the correct term to the definition.

1. ____ An anticancer treatment.

2. ____ Cross-sectional images along a single axis of the body or body structure created by a computer from multiple x-ray images.

3. ____ Enlargement of a lymph node.

4. ____ Examination of the esophagus, stomach, and duodenum using a flexible tube with scope.

5. ____ A return of symptoms or relapse.

A. CT Scan

B. recurrence

C. adenopathy

D. CHOP

E. endoscopy

THERAPEUTIC RADIOLOGY REPORT 4

PATIENT PROFILE: A 45-year-old male with stage IB adenocarcinoma of the prostate, status post primary radiation therapy for a total dose of 64.8 gray completed June 2005.

HISTORY: Mr. Smith presents today for his routine followup 2 years and 6 months after completion of radiation therapy. He continues to feel reasonably well, although he is having persistent problems with fatigue. He has recently begun using a CPAP mask for sleeping at night for his apparent sleep apnea. He continues to work full time for the post office. He denies any bone pain, has had no bowel or bladder symptoms or other constitutional symptoms.

PHYSICAL EXAMINATION: In general, this is a well-appearing, middle-aged male. He is alert and oriented. Rectal: Digital examination of the rectum reveals a smooth, firm prostate without focal nodularity and intact medial and lateral sulci.

DIAGNOSTIC STUDIES: Previous studies from his last visit in June 2007 revealed a normal CBC, normal liver function tests except for a slightly elevated ALT at 52, which has been chronic. PSA was 0.6. Chest x-ray revealed some left ventricular hypertrophy, but no evidence of metastatic disease. Bone scan showed no evidence of bony metastatic disease.

IMPRESSION: No evidence of recurrent disease.

PLAN

1. The patient is to have PSA done today.
2. He is to schedule routine followup visit in 6 months.

SPELLING.
Determine if the following words are spelled correctly. If the spelling is correct, leave the word as it has already been entered. If the spelling is incorrect, provide the correct spelling.

1. hypetrophy _____

2. prostate _____

3. persistant _____

4. apnia _____

5. nodulerity _____

TRUE/FALSE.
Mark the following true or false.

1. The patient has no current evidence of disease.

    ○ true

    ○ false

2. The patient underwent radiation therapy 6 months prior to this visit.

    ○ true

    ○ false

3. The patient uses an air machine for his sleep apnea.

    ○ true

    ○ false

4. The patient's physical exam showed no focal abnormalities.

    ○ true

    ○ false

5. A PSA is a urine test.

    ○ true

    ○ false

THERAPEUTIC RADIOLOGY REPORT 5

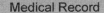

DIAGNOSIS: Stage IIIC ovarian adenocarcinoma (poorly differentiated), status post chemotherapy and maximal debulking. Now with minimal disease.

PROPOSED TREATMENT: Ms. Doe is a 53-year-old female who has undergone maximal debulking surgery for ovarian cancer recently. Prior to her surgery she did have 7 cycles of cisplatin and Cytoxan. The patient has minimal residual disease and did have involved periaortic lymph nodes. I feel the patient is a candidate for whole abdominal and pelvic irradiation. The patient would receive 2500 centigray in 25 fractions to the whole abdomen and pelvis. The kidney dose would be kept below 1800 centigray. Concurrent with this the patient would receive 80 centigray more a day to the periaortic and the pelvic lymph nodes. This would give a total dosage to the whole abdomen of 2500 centigray, and 4500 centigray to the pelvis and the periaortics. Consideration of a boost of the pelvis to 5000 centigray, plus or minus a boost to the aortics, will be contemplated. The patient may have significant toxicity from this, and the treatment plan may have to be altered substantially. The severe risks of this therapy, to include bowel obstruction, inanition, and death, have been explained to the patient and her daughter to their satisfaction.

PAST MEDICAL HISTORY: The patient does not have any major medical problems. Her surgical history includes an appendectomy at age 12, a lipoma removed from the left neck in the past, and 2 benign breast biopsies.

GYNECOLOGICAL HISTORY: The patient is gravida 3, para 3. She did not use hormones for any significant period of time. She did go through menopause at 43 years of age.

SOCIAL HISTORY: The patient is a widow and lives in Texas. She has a daughter who lives in Arkansas, and a son who lives in Nevada.[1]

FAMILY HISTORY: Brother died of cancer of the pancreas, and sister died of breast cancer.

HISTORY OF PRESENT ILLNESS: Ms. Doe is a 53-year-old female who was evaluated by Dr. Colon for gallbladder symptoms. The patient was found to have 2 inguinal hernias and did undergo exploratory laparotomy. At that time the left ovary was removed, and biopsies were taken of suspicious regions. In addition, a cholecystectomy was performed. The pathology showed that there was a poorly differentiated cyst involving the left ovary. In addition, there was biopsy-proven involvement of the omentum and the surface of the liver. Following this, the patient did receive 7 cycles of cisplatin and Cytoxan. The patient was not able to tolerate an eighth course of chemotherapy because of poor blood counts. The patient underwent total abdominal hysterectomy, right salpingo-oophorectomy, retroperitoneal lymph node dissection, and omentectomy. At that time the patient underwent maximal tumor debulking. She was found to have positive periaortic nodes. A small amount of nodal disease could not be removed, and is residual. The patient was referred for the consideration of radiotherapy.

IMPRESSION: Patient status post maximal surgical debulking and chemotherapy for a very aggressive ovarian cancer. I feel that whole abdominal radiotherapy with pelvic and periaortic boost may control this patient's disease. The mortality and morbidity of this procedure is significant and was carefully discussed with the patient and her daughter, as well as the fact that this tumor is very aggressive and is frequently incurable with the radiotherapy.

Footnotes:

1. 1.As always, the names, dates, and places are completely fictitious.

SPELLING.
Determine if the following words are spelled correctly. If the spelling is correct, leave the word as it has already been entered. If the spelling is incorrect, provide the correct spelling.

1. debulkining _____

2. peraaortic _____

3. cisplatin _____

4. chematherapy _____

5. Cytoxan

MATCHING.

Match the correct term to the definition.

1. ____ Removing the uterine tube and ovary by surgical procedure.

2. ____ Partial or total excision of the omentum.

3. ____ Treatment of disease in the abdomen by exposure to radiation.

4. ____ Removing the gallbladder by surgical procedure.

5. ____ Surgery performed to examine and/or visualize the abdomen.

A. salpingo-oophorectomy

B. cholecystectomy

C. exploratory laparotomy

D. abdominal radiotherapy

E. omentectomy

UNIT 5
Pathology

PATHOLOGY – INTRODUCTION

When you watch television these days, some of the many facets of both gross and microscopic pathology can be found on shows like *CSI*, *Homicide: Life on the Street*, and *Monk*. No doubt, even if you aren't a fan of television crime shows, in your channel surfing you've spotted an image of someone looking into a microscope, viewing a slide, hovering over a body at the morgue, or talking about organ harvesting. Pathology as a medical specialty can be broken down into two groups: anatomical and clinical pathology. Anatomic pathology deals with the gross and microscopic changes caused by disease in human cells and tissues. Clinical pathology deals with bodily fluid and waste product examination at the laboratory; specimens such as blood, urine, CSF fluid, and feces are all such products.

There are three main foci of study in pathology reports you will encounter within this unit:

- Histologic – Tissue.
- Cytologic – Cells.
- Autopsies – Postmortem examination, generally to determine cause of death.

Pathology reports, in general, are edited by pathology transcription editors; however, some basic pathology reports might be edited in the clinic and acute care settings.

PATHOLOGY LANGUAGE

Pathology as a medical specialty covers everything from developmental and growth disorders to cancer to biopsies and aspirations. Of course, what this means to you as a medical transcription editor is that the world of pathology has a language all its own. The diagnostic process itself explores tumors, cysts, tissues, exudates, hemorrhage, and homogenicity. This is a very expansive and highly technical but fascinating field which is well worth understanding in your medical transcription editor training. You may never gaze into the lens of a microscope in an effort to determine if a bloody footprint matches that of a shoe worn by the suspected killer, but you will most certainly edit pathology reports on some level. The pathology language workshop we are including in this unit is likely way more information than you need to do basic pathology reports —but it is such cool information, we are sharing it anyway! You can never have too much info, right?

PATHOLOGY LANGUAGE WORKSHOP

There are a host of samples that are sent to "the lab," by doctors and clinicians. Undoubtedly, you will be editing laboratory terminology in your career as an MTE. It would, therefore, help you to know what some of these samples mean.

Pathology Samples

Term	Definition
biopsy	Removing tissue from a living patient.
excisional biopsy	Removal of entire tumor, lesion, or affected diseased organ from a living patient.
incisional biopsy	Surgical removal of a part or section of a tumor, diseased organ, or lesion.
punch biopsy	Removal of a plug of skin or mucous membrane with a device called a "punch."
shave biopsy	Removal of a thin skin layer with a blade.
curettage	Surgical scraping.
needle biopsy	Removing inner core of tissue, such as liver and kidney.
Pap smear	Cells are detached from a surface (primarily the uterine cervix).
fine-needle aspiration (FNA)	Removing cells via suction from a mass.
washing	Using saline or other fluid to collect cells (from, for example, the stomach).
frozen section	Rapid freezing of water in tissue and embedding with paraffin or other artificial medium.

Tissue changes are at the heart of what a pathologist does. Microscopic changes can be seen in the way tissue metabolizes, grows, degenerates, and/or is impaired. Below are some terms you might encounter regarding gross and functional impairment of tissue.

Tissue Changes

Term	Definition
atrophy	Decrease in tissue bulk or structure from its previous size.
cachexia	Wasting or atrophy due to starvation.
senile atrophy	Irreversible chemical changes due to aging.
disease atrophy	Results from prolonged immobilization or lack of movement.
degeneration	Broad term in pathology referring to changes in tissue chemistry.
fatty infiltration	Fat content increases in connective tissue areas of various organs.
cholesterol	Fatty material normally found in blood but also occurring in certain tissues and diseases.
dystrophic calcification	Calcium deposits in inflamed tissue, fibrotic or degenerative tissue.
ossification	Pathologic calcification as well as bone tissue formation.
uric acid	Found in gout tissues and other metabolic disorders.
bilirubin	Bile pigment resulting from degradation of hemoglobin in the liver.
jaundice	Yellow or greenish color in tissue as a result of liver disease.
necrosis	Physical and chemical changes of tissue, cells, or organs which is seen in death.
gangrene	Local and extensive necrosis usually affecting an extremity.
infarction	Necrosis that is localized and due to an obstruction.
putrefaction	Also called decay (of the body after death).

Many of the pathologic samples and specimens submitted to "the lab" deal with terms you might have heard in other units of study in this course. However, repetition is key in sustaining your knowledge base. Every body system has its own host of pathologic specimens and disease processes. Here, we will name but a smattering, for your perusal.

Specimens and Diseases

Specimen/Disease Process	Body System/Part Affected
macule	skin
papule	skin
keloid	skin
intraductal papilloma	breast
polycystic kidney	excretory
hypernephroma	excretory
CIN (cervical intraepithelial neoplasia)	female reproductive
hydatidiform mole	female reproductive
hydrocele	male reproductive
congenital adrenal hyperplasia	endocrine
Hodgkin disease	lymph
atelectasis	respiratory
berylliosis	respiratory
ileus	digestive
peptic ulcer	digestive
staphyloma	special senses (eye)
syringomyelia	nervous
osteochondroma	skeletal
rickets	skeletal
fistula	digestive

Clinical pathology, as you know from earlier reading, deals with blood and other bodily fluids. There are many branches dealing with clinical pathology. A few of those branches, as well as some clinical terms you might hear as a medical transcription editor, are outlined below.

Common Pathology Terms

Term	Definition
hematology	Study of blood.
biochemistry	Study of chemical properties and substances which interact with the living body.
urinology	Microscopic and chemical examination of urinary specimens.
microbiology	Study of microscopic living things, such as fungi and bacteria.
diagnostic test	For disease clarification.
screening test	Used to identify disease or problems before further harm.
light microscopy	Brings out features otherwise not seen in specimens.
panel	Tests frequently performed as a group.
false positive	Positive result in an unaffected person.
false negative	Normal or negative result despite disease presence in a person.
specificity	Refers to a test's ability to reflect a specific abnormality.
reproducibility	Ability of a test to yield the same result time and again.
assay	Any quantitative test.
reagent	Chemical substance which is made to react with another substance (such as on a urine dipstick).
WNL	Within normal limits.
QNS	Quantity not sufficient.

We cannot discuss pathology without a mention of the study of blood. A chart of some hematologic terms is outlined below. You might have heard some of these terms in other units of study in this program, but they are presented here since they are an integral part of the pathologic workshop.

Hematologic/Cytologic Terms

Term	Definition
CBC (complete blood count)	Simply stated, measures red blood cells, white blood cells, and platelets.
hemoglobin	The protein in red cells that carries oxygen.
hematocrit	The proportion of blood that consists of red blood cells.
MCV (mean corpuscular volume)	Measurement of average size of RBCs.
MCH (mean corpuscular hemoglobin)	Measurement of average amount of hemoglobin inside a red blood cell.
differential	Summary of various types of white cells in a stained smear of blood.
platelet count	Test to determine how many platelets (to clot blood) in the blood.
electrolyte	Minerals of the body which have an electrical charge and are found in blood, urine.
ESR (erythrocyte sedimentation rate, sed rate)	Blood test to determine inflammation in the body.
GGT	Test to screen for liver disease, alcohol abuse.
C. diff (Clostridium difficile)	Test for bacterial toxin in feces.
BNP	Cardiac marker for heart failure.
TORCH panel	Screening for birth defects in infants and other ailments in adults.
sweat chloride test	To screen for cystic fibrosis.
CA-125	Ovarian cancer screening to determine treatment.
RF (rheumatoid factor)	To assess for rheumatoid arthritis.

REVIEW: PATHOLOGY LANGUAGE

MATCHING.
Match the correct term to the definition.

1. ____ Yellowing of the skin from liver disease.

2. ____ Physical and/or chemical changes of tissues in death.

3. ____ Surgical scraping.

4. ____ Removal of tissue from a living patient.

5. ____ Necrosis of an extremity.

6. ____ Removal of cells via suction.

7. ____ Decay after death.

8. ____ Atrophy from starvation.

9. ____ Fatty material in blood.

10. ____ Using saline to collect cells.

A. cachexia

B. curettage

C. FNA

D. gangrene

E. putrefaction

F. jaundice

G. cholesterol

H. washing

I. biopsy

J. necrosis

MULTIPLE CHOICE.
Choose the appropriate bodily system for the condition given.

1. keloid
   - ○ skin
   - ○ respiratory

2. rickets
   - ○ skeletal
   - ○ cardiovascular

3. staphyloma
   - ○ eye/special senses
   - ○ digestive

4. macule
   - ○ excretory
   - ○ skin

5. hydrocele
   - ○ female reproductive
   - ○ male reproductive

TRUE/FALSE.
Mark the following true or false.

1. Hematology is the study of urine.

   ○ true

   ○ false

2. A panel is generally performed as a group.

   ○ true

   ○ false

3. WNL means within negative limits.

   ○ true

   ○ false

4. Specificity is any quantitative test.

   ○ true

   ○ false

5. A reagent is a gaseous substance used in lab testing.

   ○ true

   ○ false

SPELLING.
Determine if the following words are spelled correctly. If the spelling is correct, leave the word as it has already been entered. If the spelling is incorrect, provide the correct spelling.

1. Clostridium dificile _____

2. differential _____

3. electrolyte _____

4. reproduceibility _____

5. microscopy _____

6. berylliosis _____

7. atelactasis _____

8. ossification _____

9. hypernephrama _____

10. erythrocyte sedementation _____

PATHOLOGY REPORTS

The following pathology reports include individual studies of various tissues or parts of the body and autopsy reports. Pathology reports consist of overall (gross) descriptions, microscopic descriptions, and diagnoses of various biopsies—such as a liver or breast biopsy, tonsils and adenoids, pieces of bones that were removed, products of conception, gallbladders, appendices, or any other structure removed from the body.

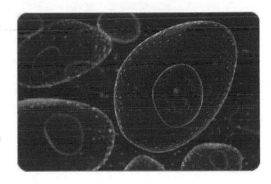

In an effort to be organized, we will group the histology/cytology pathology reports by general location in the body. Because pathology reports are descriptive in nature and cover various structures and tissues, the terminology can be very specific. However, most words in pathology are used in all types of reports and are used so often that you should find them easy to learn and remember.

PATHOLOGY REPORTS 1–3

BRIEF HISTORY: Symptomatic cholelithiasis.[1]

GROSS DESCRIPTION: Specimen is received in formalin[2] in a bag labeled "gallbladder and contents." Gallbladder is already opened and measures 9.5 x 2 x 1.5 cm. The mucosa is granular. A green, round calculus is present, 2.5 cm in diameter. A section of the gallbladder wall is submitted.

MICROSCOPIC: The wall of the gallbladder is mildly sprinkled with lymphocytes.

DIAGNOSIS: Gallbladder: chronic mild cholecystitis, cholelithiasis.

Footnotes:

1. 1.Histories will not always be given with pathology reports.
2. 2.Formalin is a solution you will hear dictated quite frequently in pathology reports. It is a 10% solution of formaldehyde in water and is used to preserve specimens for analysis.

SPECIMEN: Appendix.

GROSS DESCRIPTION: Received is a vermiform appendix which measures 8 cm in length. The serosal surface is roughened and brownish-black. All tissue is submitted as A–F.[1]

MICROSCOPIC: Histologic sections of the appendix show acute and chronic periappendicitis characterized by a mixed acute and chronic inflammatory infiltrate on the serosal surface associated with hemorrhage, vascular congestion, and edema. Sections of the appendiceal mucosa fail to show any evidence of appendicitis, as there is no acute inflammatory infiltrate involving the mucosa or the muscularis. Appropriate clinical evaluation may be needed to determine the source of the serosal inflammation.

DIAGNOSIS: Acute and chronic periappendicitis. See remarks.

Footnotes:

1. 1.Meaning the specimens are labeled A through F.

SPECIMEN:

[1]

1. Duodenal bulb.
2. Gastric.

GROSS DESCRIPTION

1. The specimen is labeled "duodenal bulb" and consists of 2 biopsies, 0.3 cm in the largest dimension. Both are submitted in block A, submitted sandwiched between foam sponges.
2. The specimen is labeled "gastric" and consists of 4 biopsies ranging between 0.2 and 0.3 cm in the largest dimension. All are submitted in block B, submitted sandwiched between foam sponges.

MICROSCOPIC

1. The sections include fragments of duodenal mucosa with villous formation on the surface. Groups of Brunner glands are seen in the adjacent submucosa. The mucosal stroma has diffuse slight chronic inflammation.
2. The sections contain fragments of gastric mucosa with glands of normal size and shape. There are focal superficial areas of ulceration as well as focal areas of superficial hemorrhage. The mucosal stroma has diffuse moderate chronic inflammation. A couple of biopsies include muscularis mucosa.

Stain for Helicobacter: No Helicobacter-like organisms are seen in part A. Seagull shaped organisms are seen on the mucosal surface in part B. The control is positive.

DIAGNOSIS

1. Slight chronic duodenitis.
2. Chronic gastritis. Helicobacter-like organisms are present.

Footnotes:

1. 1.Some accounts may prefer these be labeled 1 and 2, as opposed to A and B. There are a number of ways this could be done correctly.

SPELLING.
Determine if the following words are spelled correctly. If the spelling is correct, leave the word as it has already been entered. If the spelling is incorrect, provide the correct spelling.

1. musculairs _____

2. duadenal _____

3. superficial _____

4. inflamation _____

5. infaltrate _____

MULTIPLE CHOICE.

Choose the correct spelling for the term defined.

1. A genus of gram-negative bacteria.

   ○ Helobacter

   ○ Helicobacter

   ○ Helcobacter

   ○ Heliobacter

2. The mucous lining of various structures.

   ○ mucosa

   ○ mucousa

   ○ mucusa

   ○ moucusa

3. Covered with fine hairs.

   ○ villus

   ○ vilious

   ○ villis

   ○ villous

4. A preserving or disinfecting solution.

   ○ formlin

   ○ formelin

   ○ formalin

   ○ foramlin

5. Membranous lining of the walls of various body cavities.

   ○ serrosa

   ○ sarasa

   ○ serosa

   ○ serasa

PATHOLOGY REPORTS 4–5

BRIEF HISTORY: Inflammatory changes on Pap.[1]

GROSS DESCRIPTION

1. The specimen is labeled "ECC"[2] and consists of several red-brown mucous tissue fragments aggregating 0.4 x 0.3 x 0.2 cm, submitted in their entirety.
2. The specimen is labeled "ectocervical biopsy 9 o'clock" [3]and consists of several minute tissue fragments aggregating 0.2 x 0.2 x 0.1 cm, submitted in their entirety.

Microscopic performed, description omitted.[4]

DIAGNOSIS:

1. Endocervical curettings: Mucous debris and loose fragments of benign endocervical tissue.
2. Ectocervical biopsy: Inflammatory polyp.

Footnotes:

1. 1.Pap is short for Papanicolaou stain or smear.
2. 2.ECC stands for endocervical curettings. (Incidentally, curet can also be correctly spelled curette.)
3. 3.This, of course, doesn't mean that the biopsy was taken at 9 o'clock, rather that the location from where the biopsy was taken was the 9 o'clock position.
4. 4.This will sometimes be dictated simply as MPDO, although the expansion is not readily found in most reference books.

SPECIMEN: Vaginal biopsies.

GROSS DESCRIPTION: The specimen is labeled "vaginal biopsies" and consists of several tan-gray soft tissue fragments aggregating 0.3 x 0.2 x 0.2 cm and are submitted in their entirety.

MICROSCOPIC: Multiple H&E sections[1] were reviewed which show normal appearing vaginal mucosa. Underneath the vaginal mucosa are tight clusters of malignant cells which are elongated and very pleomorphic in appearance. No glandular formations are identified. There is marked necrosis seen as well as occasional bizarre mitotic figures. No keratin pearls or intracellular bridging can be identified.

DIAGNOSIS: Vaginal biopsies: Poorly-differentiated carcinoma, probably squamous cell type.

COMMENT: Although the biopsies show a very poorly-differentiated carcinoma, there are some features of a squamous cell type, and because of this, the patient should be evaluated for a primary from the genitourinary tract.

Footnotes:

1. 1.H&E sections are sections stained with haematoxylin and eosin.

SPELLING.
Determine if the following words are spelled correctly. If the spelling is correct, leave the word as it has already been entered. If the spelling is incorrect, provide the correct spelling.

1. malignent _____

2. carcenoma _____

3. aggregating _____

4. keratin _____

5. intracelular _____

MATCHING.
Match the correct term to the definition.

1. ____ A mass of tissue or vascular growth.

2. ____ Pertaining to mitosis, cell division.

3. ____ Localized death of living cells.

4. ____ Scaly or platelike.

5. ____ Having various distinct forms.

A. pleomorphic

B. necrosis

C. polyp

D. squamous

E. mitotic

PATHOLOGY REPORT 6

SPECIMEN: Cone biopsy, endocervical curettings, endometrial curettings.

GROSS DESCRIPTION

1. Received in saline in a bag labeled "cone biopsy" is a cervical cone measuring 1.3 x 2.2 x 1 cm. When opened, the circumference is 3 cm. There is no suture to indicate the 12 o'clock position on the cone. After overnight fixation, the sections of the cone are totally embedded in 3 cassettes.
2. Received in formalin in a bag labeled "endocervical curettings," on Teflon, are fragments of soft pinkish-red tissue aggregating 1 x 0.7 x 0.5 cm, totally embedded.
3. Received in formalin in a bag labeled "endometrial curettings," on Teflon, are fragments of soft hemorrhagic tissue, aggregating 1 x 1 x 0.5 cm, totally embedded.

MICROSCOPIC

1. The squamous epithelium covering the ectocervical portion of the cone is hyperplastic and shows mild koilocytotic atypia.[1] Covering the endocervical portion of the cone is columnar epithelium and in 1 or 2 sections dysplastic squamous epithelium is present, also involving the neck of a few endocervical glands. The dysplasia is characterized by cellular crowding and nuclear hyperchromatism[2] with slight pleomorphism in the basal 3/4[3] and focally involving the entire thickness of the epithelium. The basement membrane is intact. There is no dysplasia at the margins of the cone.
2. Mixed with blood and mucus are fragments of endometrium from the lower uterine segment, as well as endocervical tissue, with no squamous epithelium present.
3. Fragments of endometrium with mildly dilated glands lined by secretory columnar epithelium. Slight edema is present in the stroma. A fragment of endocervical tissue is also present showing chronic inflammation.

DIAGNOSIS

1. Cone biopsy: Focal moderate and severe dysplasia, CIN II and III[4] at the transitional zone. Squamous epithelial hyperplasia of exocervical tissue with mild koilocytotic atypia.
2. Endocervical curettings: No pathological change.
3. Endometrial curettings: Secretory endometrium.

Footnotes:

1. 1.A finding of koilocytotic atypia typically means further testing, as it can be premalignant.
2. 2.Hyperchromatism = abnormal increase in pigmentation.
3. 3.This could also be edited as "three fourths." You do not need a hyphen, although it would not necessarily be incorrect to edit it with a hyphen. The general rule is to not use a hyphen with spelled out fractions less than one unless they are followed by a noun (three fourths or three-fourths liter).
4. 4.CIN = cervical intraepithelial neoplasia.

SPELLING.
Determine if the following words are spelled correctly. If the spelling is correct, leave the word as it has already been entered. If the spelling is incorrect, provide the correct spelling.

1. epithelial _____

2. pathalogical _____

3. dialated _____

4. margins _____

5. edema _____

FILL IN THE BLANK.

Using the word(s) in the box, enter the appropriate term in the space provided.

1. Cells or tissue that have undergone abnormal development are referred to as

   _____ .

2. When a _____ biopsy is performed, a cone-shaped wedge of tissue is taken from the cervix.

3. The term _____ means external to the cervix.

4. The term _____ means pertaining to secretion.

5. The _____ covers the internal organs.

cone
dysplastic
epithelium
exocervical
secretory

PATHOLOGY REPORTS 7–9

SPECIMEN: Left and right vas, right epididymal cyst.[1]

GROSS DESCRIPTION

1. Received in formalin in a container labeled "left vas and spermatocele" is a firm tubular structure 5 mm in length and 3 mm in diameter. Also present is a cystic structure with a thin wall filled with clear fluid, measuring 2.7 x 1.5 x 1 cm. A cross section of the cyst is submitted along with the tubular structure in 1 cassette.
2. Received in formalin in a bag labeled "right vas" is a tubular structure, 5 mm in length and 3 mm in diameter, totally embedded.

MICROSCOPIC: A and B: The sections of the vas deferens are histologically normal. The wall of the cyst is thin and consists of loose connective tissue. The cyst is lined by flat epithelium. In the connective tissue, there are efferent ducts.

DIAGNOSIS

1. Histologically unremarkable segment of left vas deferens. Epididymal cyst, consistent with spermatocele. Histologically unremarkable segment of right vas deferens.

Footnotes:

1. 1.Vas as in vas deferens. And epididymal as in relating to the tube in the testis that carries sperm to the vas deferens.

SPECIMEN: Sigmoidoscopically obtained biopsy specimen.

GROSS DESCRIPTION: The specimen is labeled "22 cm colon polyp" and consists of a small piece of red tissue, 0.3 cm in its largest dimension. Submitted in toto[1]in 1 block, submitted sandwiched between foam sponges.

MICROSCOPIC: A total of 8 sections are available for microscopic examination. They all contain fragments of colonic mucosa with areas of focal intramucosal hemorrhage. Some of the glands vary in size and are partially covered by pseudostratified columnar epithelium.

DIAGNOSIS: Polyp with focal adenomatous changes and focal hemorrhage.

Footnotes:

1. 1.In toto is a fancy (or Latin) way to say "in entirety" or "as a whole."

SPECIMEN: Hidradenitis, suppurative, left groin.

GROSS DESCRIPTION: Received in formalin in a bag labeled "hidradenitis" is an ellipse of gray skin with subcutaneous tissue, 2.1 x 0.5 x 1.5 cm. Trisected and totally embedded.

MICROSCOPIC: The epidermis is slightly hyperplastic. There is fibrosis in the dermis with chronic inflammation present. A small epidermal inclusion cyst is seen filled with keratin. There are no sweat glands.

DIAGNOSIS: Skin left groin: Mild dermal fibrosis with chronic inflammation and small epidermal inclusion cyst.

SPELLING.
Determine if the following words are spelled correctly. If the spelling is correct, leave the word as it has already been entered. If the spelling is incorrect, provide the correct spelling.

1. sweet glands _____

2. fiberosis _____

3. inclusion _____

4. supurative _____

5. hidradinitis _____

MULTIPLE CHOICE.

Choose the correct spelling for the term defined.

1. An epididymal cyst.
   - ○ spermetaceale
   - ○ spermatoceale
   - ○ spermatocele
   - ○ spermitoceale

2. Closely packed cells that are all attached to the basement membrane, but that appear to be layered.
   - ○ pseudastratified
   - ○ pseudostratified
   - ○ pseudostratefied
   - ○ pseudalstratified

3. Pertaining to a nodular hyperplasia of a gland.
   - ○ adenomatous
   - ○ adanomatus
   - ○ adinomatous
   - ○ addenomatous

4. An oval or oblong shape.
   - ○ ellipse
   - ○ elipse
   - ○ eclipse
   - ○ alipse

5. Fibrous scleroprotein occurring in the outer layer of skin, hair, nails, etc.
   - ○ keratin
   - ○ karatin
   - ○ keritin
   - ○ keretin

SPECIMEN: Placenta

GROSS DESCRIPTION: Received in formalin in a container labeled with the patient's name is the placenta, 16 x 14 x 2.5 cm. The point of nearest rupture of the membrane is 3 cm from the edge of the placenta. The umbilical cord is centrally attached, and the cord measures 35 cm in length and 1 cm in diameter. On the maternal side, cotyledons[1] are intact. A few thin clots are adherent to the placenta on the maternal side. Without the cord and membranes, the placenta weighs 330 grams. Sections of the placenta, cord, and membrane were submitted in 5 cassettes.

MICROSCOPIC: The chorionic villi are small and well vascularized. No areas of hemorrhage or necrosis seen. There is no gross or microscopic evidence of abruption. The chorionic plate and fetal membranes show no inflammation. The umbilical cord contains 2 arteries and 1 vein.

DIAGNOSIS: Placenta, cord, membranes, no pathological change.

Footnotes:

1. 1. A cotyledon is any portion of the uterine surface of the placenta.

SPECIMEN: Conception products with placenta, 20 week IUP.[1]

GROSS DESCRIPTION: The specimen consists of a placenta with attached umbilical cord and fetus. The fetus weighs 186 grams. No gross external abnormalities are noted. The abdomen appears to be slightly distended. The external genitalia are of male type. The internal viscera appear to be normally situated and related. No gross abnormalities. The liver weighs 14 grams. Both lungs and liver are sampled in block #1. The umbilical cord is 16 cm in length and is inserted at the edge of the placental disc. The membranes are opaque and appear to be complete. The placental disc, trimmed of membranes and umbilical cord, weighs 136 grams. The placental tissue has some areas of tawny mottling on the maternal surface. No gross abnormalities noted on multiple cross sections. Representative sections submitted in 2 blocks.

MICROSCOPIC: The fetal lung has normal histology. The fetal liver has extensive erythropoiesis which is to be expected. Also noted is marked congestion of the liver tissue. The placental tissue has numerous syncytial knots. The umbilical cord has three blood vessels. The membranes have acute inflammation.

DIAGNOSIS: Products of conception. Acute chorioamnionitis.[2]

Footnotes:

1. 1. IUP = intrauterine pregnancy
2. 2. Chorioamnionitis, as breaking down the word will show you, means inflammation of the chorion and amnion.

SPELLING.
Determine if the following words are spelled correctly. If the spelling is correct, leave the word as it has already been entered. If the spelling is incorrect, provide the correct spelling.

1. conception _____

2. vesels _____

3. placenta _____

4. choroinic villi _____

5. histrology _____

MATCHING.
Match the correct term to the definition.

1. ____ Formation of red blood cells.

2. ____ Any portion of the uterine surface of the placenta.

3. ____ Pertaining to the mass of protoplasm created when cells merge.

4. ____ Death of living cells.

5. ____ Bleeding; blood flowing from vessels.

A. syncytial

B. hemorrhage

C. necrosis

D. erythropoiesis

E. cotyledon

PATHOLOGY REPORTS 12–13

SPECIMEN: Breast biopsy.

GROSS DESCRIPTION: The specimen is labeled "left breast biopsy with needle localization" and consists of several fresh fibroadipose tissue fragments which in aggregate measure 3.8 x 2.5 x 1.4 cm. The portion of tissue which shows radiographic calcifications is submitted in cassette #1, and the remainder of the specimen is submitted in cassettes 2–4.

Microscopic performed, description omitted.

DIAGNOSIS: Left breast biopsy: sclerosing adenosis and dermofibrosis.

SPECIMEN: Right breast mass; left breast mole.

GROSS DESCRIPTION

1. PART A: The specimen is labeled "right breast mass, fresh" and consists of a firm fresh fibroadipose tissue specimen aggregating 2.8 x 2.1 x 1.5 cm. As the specimen is serially sectioned, several areas are noted to have a very gritty, firm appearance. A representative section is frozen for receptor studies. The remainder of the specimen is submitted in its entirety in cassettes A1-4.
2. The specimen is labeled "left breast mole" and consists of 1 gray-tan soft tissue fragment which in aggregate measures 0.4 x 0.3 x 0.3 cm. The specimen is bisected and submitted in its entirety in 1 cassette.

MICROSCOPIC

1. Multiple H&E sections were reviewed which showed neoplasm composed of glandular cribriform-like[1] structures. The cells making up the cribriform structures are pleomorphic, hyperchromatic, showing occasional minute nucleoli. These malignant cells are not only in clusters, but are seen to infiltrate surrounding stromal tissue, and in single-file infiltration. A desmoplastic[2] reaction is noted with the neoplasm.

   The histologic sections show dermal fibrosis and edema.

DIAGNOSIS:

1. Right breast mass: Infiltrating ductal carcinoma.
2. Left breast mole, excision: Dermal fibrosis and edema.

Footnotes:

1. 1. Cribriform essentially means pierced with holes, like a sieve.
2. 2. If you are not sure what desmoplastic means, make sure to look it up! This is a good one to add to your word list.

SPELLING.
Determine if the following words are spelled correctly. If the spelling is correct, leave the word as it has already been entered. If the spelling is incorrect, provide the correct spelling.

1. dermil _____
2. neoplasm _____
3. entirty _____
4. speciman _____
5. fibradipose _____

MULTIPLE CHOICE.
Choose the best answer.

1. To gather in a mass is to (○ aggregate, ○ aggregate).
2. The formation and development of fibrous tissue is referred to as (○ desmoplasia, ○ dermoplasia).
3. Something which passes into or permeates through is said to be (○ infitrating, ○ infiltrating).
4. The placement of something is determined during (○ localization, ○ localazation).
5. When something is deemed (○ hypochromatic, ○ hyperchromatic), it shows more than normal staining.

PATHOLOGY REPORTS 14–16

SPECIMEN: Adenoids, right and left tonsils.

GROSS DESCRIPTION

1. Received in formalin in a bag labeled "adenoids" is a piece of soft pink tissue consistent with adenoids, 2.2 x 1.5 x 1 cm. Sections are totally embedded in 1 cassette.
2. Received in formalin in a bag labeled "right and left tonsils" are 2 slightly lobulated tonsils, each measuring 3 x 2 x 1.5 cm. One section of each tonsil submitted in 1 cassette.

MICROSCOPIC:

A & B: In the lymphoid tissue of the adenoids and tonsils are many large follicles with prominent germinal centers. The adenoids are covered by columnar epithelium. The squamous epithelium of the tonsils is benign, and in the crypts,[1]inflammatory debris is present.

DIAGNOSIS: A & B: Follicular hyperplasia of the tonsils and adenoids.

Footnotes:

1. 1.If you are a visual person, you probably envision tonsillar crypts to be something like clefts or cave-like recessions in the tonsils. You would be right!

SPECIMEN: Biopsy from tongue.

GROSS DESCRIPTION: Received in formalin in a container labeled "right lateral border of tongue" is a fragment of gray-white tissue, 5 x 4 x 3 mm, totally embedded.

MICROSCOPIC: The surface squamous epithelium is benign, although hyperplastic, forming elongated rete ridges[1] with parakeratosis on the surface.

DIAGNOSIS: Squamous epithelial hyperplasia with parakeratosis.

Footnotes:

1. 1.If you look up rete ridges, you will see that they are the downward thickening of the epidermis between the dermal papillae. (If you aren't sure what dermal papillae means, look it up.)

SPECIMEN: Scar and cartilage, right ear, postauricular.

GROSS DESCRIPTION: Received in formalin in a bag labeled "cartilage and scar" are 2 fragments of pink tissue aggregating 1.5 x 1.3 x 0.7 cm, totally embedded.

MICROSCOPIC: One fragment consists of dense collagen fibrous tissue consistent with scar with a small amount of fat tissue present. The second specimen consists of a piece of mature cartilage.

DIAGNOSIS: Scar tissue and cartilage, right ear, postauricular.

SPELLING.
Determine if the following words are spelled correctly. If the spelling is correct, leave the word as it has already been entered. If the spelling is incorrect, provide the correct spelling.

1. cartilage _____

2. fragament _____

3. embedded _____

4. lataral _____

5. formlin _____

MATCHING.
Match the correct term to the definition.

1. ____ Situated to the back of the ear.

2. ____ Pathology seen in psoriasis.

3. ____ The major protein of white fibers of cartilage, bone, and connective tissues.

4. ____ Injured tissue that has healed and has a fibrous cover.

5. ____ A spherical mass of cells.

A. scar

B. postauricular

C. follicle

D. collagen

E. parakeratosis

PATHOLOGY REPORT 17

AUTOPSY REPORT[1]

PRELIMINARY PATHOLOGICAL DIAGNOSES
LUNGS

1. Fibrosis upper lobes.
2. Pleural adhesions with obliteration of pleural spaces.

ADRENALS: Granulomas
BLADDER: Cystitis.

FINAL ANATOMIC DIAGNOSES
AORTA: Atherosclerosis, mild, aortic arch.
LUNGS

1. Fibrosis apical lobes with caseating granulomas.[2]
2. Pleural adhesions with obliteration of pleural spaces.

LIVER: Fatty liver, marked.
CEREBELLUM: Subarachnoid hemorrhage, right cerebellum, slight.
BLADDER: Cystitis, mild.

CLINICAL SUMMARY: This 59-year-old male patient was found unconscious with no pulse and no respirations by paramedics in the bathroom on March 11. He had no history of heart problems. He was immediately intubated, resuscitated, 3 times defibrillated, and rushed to the emergency room where CPR was continued for another 25 minutes. The patient showed no response and was pronounced dead. His past medical history included active pulmonary TB, adrenal insufficiency and possible Addison disease in 1998, on cortisone acetate 25 mg tablets. The last admission to hospital was in December for acute alcohol intoxication, alcoholic hypoglycemia, and possible aspiration pneumonia.

GROSS EXAMINATION: The body for examination is that of a well-developed, elderly male, identified by the name of John Doe by means of a name tag tied around the left great toe. Rigor mortis has set in. The scalp is nontraumatic. The scalp hair is thick, grayish-black. A linear suture in a vertical cut is seen over the right eyebrow, 3.5 cm in length. The eyes are somewhat sunken, and the corneae are slightly cloudy with arcus senilis present. The pupils are dilated 5 mm on both sides. Sclerae are nonicteric[3] and conjunctivae are pale. Ears and nose are not remarkable. In the mouth an endotracheal tube is still in place. A yellowish streak of bile staining is noted at the corner of the mouth on the right side. The face is unshaved. The neck is cylindrical, and the chest is symmetrical. A crusty, light brown area of the skin in the midsternum is seen, 3.5 x 2.5 cm. Needle puncture marks are present in the left antecubital fossa, and there is a venous line in the left wrist. The abdomen is flat. The penis is uncircumcised. There is no edema in the lower extremities. The back and anus are unremarkable.

A "Y" shaped incision is made to open the body. The subcutaneous fat in the midline is 2 cm thick. There is no fluid in the peritoneal cavity. The pleural spaces are totally obliterated by pleural adhesions, and the lungs can be removed only with great difficulty.

Both lungs combined weigh 1200 grams. The apical portions of the upper lobes of the lungs are almost solid from fibrosis. Other lobes of the lungs are minimally inflated, but no masses are present. No thromboemboli in the pulmonary vessels, and no lesions in the bronchi/bronchioli.

In the pericardial space, the usual small amount of pericardial fluid is present. The heart weighs 350 grams. Cardiac valves are grossly unremarkable with the following circumferences: Aortic valve 8 cm, pulmonic valve 9 cm, tricuspid valve 12 cm, mitral valve 8.5 cm. Coronary arteries are patent. The heart muscle is beefy-red throughout.

The aorta shows no significant atherosclerotic changes. Some calcified yellowish plaque formation is noted in the aortic arch.

The liver is 1350 grams. The serosal surface is smooth. Cut surfaces of the liver are light brown and homogeneous. The gallbladder is 11 x 5 x 3 cm, filled with bile. No stones present.

The spleen weighs 45 grams. The organ is dark purple, and parenchyma is reddish purple.

The GI tract shows no erosions or ulcerations. The appendix is 8 cm in length and 0.6 cm in diameter. No diverticula in the sigmoid colon. The pancreas is of normal size and shape, and the parenchyma shows the usual lobular glandular appearance.

The adrenals weigh 8 and 6 grams. The cut sections are grayish-white without showing the usual distinction of cortex and medulla. In the left adrenal is a soft grayish nodule occupying most of the cut surface.

The right and left kidneys weigh respectively 220 and 240 grams. The thin fibrous capsules strip with no difficulty, revealing a fairly smooth pink-gray cortical surface. Cut sections of the kidneys show a clear demarcation of the cortex and striated medulla. There is no dilation of the pelves or ureters.

The bladder contains a very small amount of thick, cloudy, gray-white material. The mucosa of the bladder is wrinkled. The prostate is 4 x 3.5 x 3 cm without nodularities.

The skull is opened and the brain removed. No subdural/subarachnoid or intracerebral hemorrhage is noted. The brain weighs 1220 grams. Hemispheres are symmetrical. At the base of the brain, the arteries show no significant sclerotic changes. The unci are not prominent. There is no grooving at the cerebellar tonsils. On the right side, a small clot covers the cerebellar folia. Coronal sections of the brain show symmetrical lateral ventricles. No masses or hemorrhage seen in the cerebrum, cerebellum, or brainstem. The following sections are submitted for microscopic exam:

1. Right central cortex.
2. Left hippocampus.
3. Right corpus striatum.
4. Mid brain.
5. Right cerebellum.
6. Left cerebellum.

PRELIMINARY PATHOLOGICAL DIAGNOSES
HEART: The heart muscle is histologically unremarkable.
LUNGS: Sections of the apical portions of the lungs show dense fibrosis with scattered caseating granulomas present. Stains for AFB and fungi are negative (controls are positive). Capillaries are dilated and congested. Sections of other lobes of the lung show vascular congestion.
LIVER: Marked fatty change of the liver involving almost all cells in the liver lobules. A mild sprinkling with lymphocytes is noted in some portal tracts. No cirrhosis.
SPLEEN: Histologically within normal limits.
PANCREAS: Focal autolysis noted.
ADRENALS: Adrenal structure is almost obliterated by fibrosis with hyalinization or caseating granulomas present. Only scattered tiny nests of adrenal cortical cells remain. AFB and fungal stains negative.
KIDNEYS: Histologically within normal limits.
BLADDER: Mucosa is mildly sprinkled with lymphocytes.
PROSTATE: Histologically normal.
CNS: Dropout of Purkinje cells and ganglion cells in the dentate nucleus of the cerebellum noted. There is slight subarachnoid hemorrhage over the right cerebellum. No significant pathologic change is noted in other sections of the brain or brain stem.

CLINICOPATHOLOGIC CORRELATION: This 59-year-old male was found unconscious without pulse and respirations in the bathroom. Resuscitation was begun immediately by paramedics, and he was rushed to the emergency room. He was virtually dead upon arrival. Resuscitation was continued for another 25 minutes with no response from the patient.

Postmortem examination revealed a markedly fatty liver compatible with a history of chronic alcoholism. A significant finding was the fibrosed adrenals containing hyalinized and caseating granulomas, confirming the diagnosis of Addison disease. The adrenal insufficiency could have caused an episode of hypoglycemia and unconsciousness and ultimately death. The patient sustained only a little trauma from his fall: a small cut over the right eyebrow, and a small hemorrhage over the right cerebrum. Caseating granulomas in the fibrosed apical lobes of the lungs were also consistent with a history of tuberculosis.

Footnotes:

1. 1.Unless you work specifically for a hospital pathology department or morgue, you will not likely edit autopsy reports. You may, however, edit your fair share of death summaries if you work in an acute care setting.
2. 2.To caseate is to become "cheeselike" or have the appearance of whitish necrotic material.
3. 3.The term "nonicteric" is commonly used to mean without jaundice. The more correct word is anicteric and "back in the day" it was generally preferred MTEs change nonicteric to anicteric, even when dictated. Today, however, it is generally preferred to edit the word as dictated. The meaning is clear either way.

SPELLING.
Determine if the following words are spelled correctly. If the spelling is correct, leave the word as it has already been entered. If the spelling is incorrect, provide the correct spelling.

1. casaeting _____

2. postmorten _____

3. resusitation _____

4. adrennals _____

5. histologically _____

MULTIPLE CHOICE.

Choose the correct spelling of the term.

1. The layer of tissue between the pia mater and the arachnoid.
   - subarachnoid
   - subarachanoid
   - subrachnoid
   - subirachnoid

2. Liver disease commonly caused by alcoholism.
   - cirrosis
   - cirhosis
   - cirrhosis
   - cirhhosis

3. Postmortem change seen in cellular components.
   - autolisis
   - autolisys
   - autalysis
   - autolysis

4. Structure that houses the chromosomes.
   - nucleus
   - nucleaus
   - nuclus
   - nucleius

5. The smallest blood vessels.
   - capilaries
   - capillaries
   - capallaries
   - capalaries

ANSWER KEY

Emergency Room

REVIEW: EMERGENCY ROOM LANGUAGE

I. MULTIPLE CHOICE.
appendectomy
bleed
sedimentation

2. bicarb
4. abdominal

II. FILL IN THE BLANK.
basic
consciousness
lactated
rhythm
mortality

2. arrival
4. resuscitation
6. intravenous
8. therapy
10. range

III. TRUE/FALSE.
false
true
true

2. false
4. false

EMERGENCY ROOM REPORT 1

I. SPELLING.
Caucasian
creatinine
heme

2. appendectomy
4. murmur

II. MULTIPLE CHOICE.
expiratory
has not
afebrile

2. intravenously
4. 3

EMERGENCY ROOM REPORT 2

I. MULTIPLE CHOICE.
mandible
crepitus
deficit

2. maxilla
4. oriented

II. TRUE/FALSE.
false
true
false

2. false
4. true

EMERGENCY ROOM REPORT 3

I. SPELLING.
cardiac
Aciphex
hypertrophy

2. hemoglobin
4. epigastric

II. TRUE/FALSE.
true
false
false

2. true
4. false

EMERGENCY ROOM REPORT 4

I. FILL IN THE BLANK.

purulent
intracranial
auscultation

2. temporal
4. consciousness

II. TRUE/FALSE.

false
true
true

2. true
4. false

EMERGENCY ROOM REPORT 5

I. SPELLING.

sweating
hypokalemia
rhythm

2. tibial
4. bilaterally

II. MULTIPLE CHOICE.

palpitation
dorsal pedal
nausea

2. beta blockers
4. tachycardia

EMERGENCY ROOM REPORT 6

I. MULTIPLE CHOICE.

mucous
prostatic
anorexia

2. diarrhea
4. incontinence

II. TRUE/FALSE.

true
false
true

2. false
4. false

EMERGENCY ROOM REPORT 7

I. SPELLING.

cranial
septum
naproxen

2. scarring
4. rabeprazole

II. TRUE/FALSE.

false
false
true

2. true
4. true

EMERGENCY ROOM REPORT 8

I. MULTIPLE CHOICE.

stent
nitroglycerin
atypical

2. nondistended
4. cannula

II. MULTIPLE CHOICE.

auscultation
respiration
bllaterally

2. cardiopulmonary
4. myocardial

EMERGENCY ROOM REPORT 9

I. FILL IN THE BLANK.

depressive

otic

cerumen

2. ideation

4. adenopathy

II. MATCHING.

B. heart

A. skin

C. neck

2. E. abdomen

4. D. vital signs

REVIEW: PHYSICAL MEDICINE LANGUAGE

I. MULTIPLE CHOICE.
assisted
head
front

2. prosthetics
4. leg

II. SPELLING.
Galeazzi
dorsiflexion
caudal
immobilizer
disarticulation

2. peripheral
4. Yergason
6. tenosynovitis
8. costoclavicular
10. Lachman

III. MATCHING.
B. medial
D. inferior
A. peripheral
E. anterior
C. lateral

2. G. plantar
4. J. posterior
6. F. cranial
8. I. palmar
10. H. caudal

IV. TRUE/FALSE.
false
false
false

2. false
4. true

PHYSICAL MEDICINE REPORT 1 – CONSULTATION

I. MULTIPLE CHOICE.
ulnar
lateral
dynamometer

2. abduction
4. thumb

II. TRUE/FALSE.
true
true
false

2. false
4. false

PHYSICAL MEDICINE REPORT 2 – CONSULTATION

I. SPELLING.
ambulation
dorsiflexion
numbness

2. inversion
4. fibula

II. TRUE/FALSE.
false
true
true

2. false
4. false

PHYSICAL MEDICINE REPORT 3 – DISCHARGE SUMMARY

I. SPELLING.

weightbearing
flexion
balance

2. therapy
4. coordination

II. MULTIPLE CHOICE.

sclerosis
gait
ambulation

2. fatigues
4. ease

PHYSICAL MEDICINE REPORT 4 – CONSULTATION

I. TRUE/FALSE.

false
true
true

2. false
4. false

II. SPELLING.

cortisone
labrum
teres minor

2. intermittent
4. resistive

PHYSICAL MEDICINE REPORT 5 – CONSULTATION

I. MULTIPLE CHOICE.

posture
Phalen
Tinel

2. volar
4. epicondyle

II. TRUE/FALSE.

true
false
false

2. false
4. true

PHYSICAL MEDICINE REPORT 6 – DISCHARGE SUMMARY

I. SPELLING.

hypermobile
girth
plantar

2. avulsed
4. aerobic

II. MULTIPLE CHOICE.

motion
hallucis
foot

2. inversion
4. mobility

PHYSICAL MEDICINE REPORT 7 – CONSULTATION

I. SPELLING.

contusion
extremity
bruising

2. approximately
4. inversion

II. TRUE/FALSE.

false
false
false

2. true
4. true

PHYSICAL MEDICINE REPORT 8 – CONSULTATION

I. TRUE/FALSE.

true

false

false

2. false

4. true

II. MULTIPLE CHOICE.

course

traumatic

mobilization

2. temporomandibular

4. segmental

PHYSICAL MEDICINE REPORT 9 – CONSULTATION

I. UNSCRAMBLE.

Phalen test OR phalen

occupational OR occupational therapy

Finkelstein test OR finkelstein

Futuro wrist brace OR Futuro

2. Tinel sign OR tinel

4. Jaymar dynamometer OR dynamometer

6. carpal OR carpal tunnel therapy

8. lateral epicondylitis OR epicondylitis

Radiology

REVIEW: RADIOLOGY LANGUAGE

I. MULTIPLE CHOICE.
vertical
ureters
cystourethrogram

2. electroencephalogram
4. unequal

II. SPELLING.
proctosigmoidoscopy
roentgenology
lumbosacral

2. pyelogram
4. sagittal

III. TRUE/FALSE.
false
false
false

2. false
4. false

IV. MATCHING.
B. oblique
G. supine
A. extension
I. PA view
C. left lateral view

2. E. AP view
4. H. prone
6. F. flexion
8. J. inversion
10. D. lateral decubitus

V. MULTIPLE CHOICE.
multiple gated acquisition
single-photon emission computed tomography
posteroanterior

2. hydroxyiminodiacetic acid
4. computed tomography

BONE X-RAY REPORTS 1–3

I. SPELLING.
dorsal
fusion
avulsion

2. malleolus
4. metaphysis

II. MATCHING.
C. coronoid
D. crepitus
E. periosteal

2. A. ossicle
4. B. angulation

BONE X-RAY REPORTS 4–6

I. SPELLING.
thorax
sacroiliac
plaquing

2. prevertebral
4. osteoblastic

II. MULTIPLE CHOICE.
pneumomediastinum
diffuse idiopathic skeletal hyperostosis
diverticula

2. subluxation
4. phlebolith

BONE X-RAY REPORTS 7–9

I. SPELLING.

osteoarthritis

phalanx

lucency

2. parietal

4. osteophyte

II. MULTIPLE CHOICE.

interphalangeal

carpometacarpal

Heberden's

2. lytic

4. phalangeal

CHEST X-RAY REPORTS 1–3

I. SPELLING.

nasogastric

pleural

bilateral

2. apical

4. abnormalities

II. MULTIPLE CHOICE.

scarring

prominent

pneumonia

2. effusions

4. infiltrates

CHEST X-RAY REPORTS 4–6

I. SPELLING.

Fallot

tetralogy

granulomata

2. hypertrophy

4. thoracotomy

II. MATCHING.

E. infiltration

A. osteophyte

C. granuloma

2. D. cardiomegaly

4. B. edema

CHEST X-RAY REPORTS 7–9

I. SPELLING.

subclavian

proximal

cephalic

2. glenoid fossa OR glenoid

4. peripheral

II. MATCHING.

B. lymphangitic

D. thrombocytopenia

A. pneumothorax

2. E. iliac

4. C. superimposed

ULTRASOUND REPORTS 1–3

I. SPELLING.

caliectasis

anteroposterior

effusion

2. subpulmonic

4. hemithorax

II. MULTIPLE CHOICE.

biliary

spleen

versus

2. hydronephrosis

4. echogenicity

ULTRASOUND REPORT 4

I. SPELLING.

ventriculomegaly
occipitofrontal
intrauterine

2. femur
4. circumference

II. FILL IN THE BLANK.

menstrual
amniotic
cord

2. previa
4. intracranial

ULTRASOUND REPORT 5

I. SPELLING.

carotid
occlusion
cerebrovascular

2. fibrinous
4. systolic

II. MATCHING.

E. proximal
D. arteriosclerotic
C. antegrade

2. B. intimal
4. A. stenosis

MRI REPORTS 1–2

I. SPELLING.

facet
Magnevist
basilar

2. foraminal
4. paracentral

II. MULTIPLE CHOICE.

vertigo
plane
hypertrophy

2. osteophyte
4. multiplanar gradient recall

MRI REPORTS 3–4

I. SPELLING.

sagittal
ischemic
atrophy

2. centrum semiovale OR semiovale
4. pulposus

II. TRUE/FALSE.

false
true
false

2. true
4. true

CT SCAN REPORTS 1–2

I. SPELLING.

cortical
fossa
contiguous

2. sulci
4. clivus

II. MATCHING.

C. midline shift
E. cortical
A. myoclonic

2. B. eosinophilic granuloma
4. D. contrast

CT SCAN REPORTS 3–4

I. SPELLING.
Gastrografin
abscess
choledochojejunostomy

2. hypertrophy
4. Omnipaque

II. MULTIPLE CHOICE.
tract
flavum
reflux

2. contiguous
4. laminectomy

CONTRAST STUDY REPORTS 1–2

I. SPELLING.
calcific
esophagus
enteroclysis

2. cricopharyngeal
4. melena

II. MULTIPLE CHOICE.
arteriovenous
nonsteroidal
gastroesophageal

2. ingested
4. polyps

CONTRAST STUDY REPORTS 3–4

I. SPELLING.
spontaneously
obstruction
ascending

2. Urovist
4. redundant

II. MATCHING.
B. ureteropelvic junction
A. diverticulitis
D. voiding

2. C. cecum
4. E. reflux

CONTRAST STUDY REPORT 5

I. SPELLING.
obstruction
gastrojejunal
pancreatic

2. afferent
4. inversion

II. FILL IN THE BLANK.
efferent
anastomosis
palliative

2. celiotomy
4. fistula

MAMMOGRAPHY REPORT 1

I. SPELLING.
microcalcifications
suspicious
localization

2. quadrant
4. cyst

II. MULTIPLE CHOICE.
ovoid
thoracic
lesion

2. dense
4. distortion

MAMMOGRAPHY REPORTS 2–3

I. SPELLING.

quadrant

baseline

mastectomy

2. counseled

4. radiodense

II. MULTIPLE CHOICE.

infiltrating

morphology

architectural

2. malignancy

4. suspicious

THERAPEUTIC RADIOLOGY REPORT 1

I. SPELLING.

calcitonin

thyroidectomy

residual

2. extracapsular

4. thymic

II. FILL IN THE BLANK.

metastatic

benign

adjuvant

2. medullary

4. parathyroid

THERAPEUTIC RADIOLOGY REPORT 2

I. SPELLING.

adenocarcinoma

collimated

Cerrobend

2. hilar

4. desquamation

II. MULTIPLE CHOICE.

vena

oblique

megavolt

2. Domeboro

4. photon

THERAPEUTIC RADIOLOGY REPORT 3

I. SPELLING.

evidence

hepatosplenomegaly

radiation

2. abdominal

4. lymphatics

II. MATCHING.

D. CHOP

C. adenopathy

B. recurrence

2. A. CT Scan

4. E. endoscopy

THERAPEUTIC RADIOLOGY REPORT 4

I. SPELLING.

hypertrophy

persistent

nodularity

2. prostate

4. apnea

II. TRUE/FALSE.

true

true

false

2. false

4. true

THERAPEUTIC RADIOLOGY REPORT 5

I. SPELLING.

debulking

cisplatin

Cytoxan

2. periaortic

4. chemotherapy

II. MATCHING.

A. salpingo-oophorectomy

D. abdominal radiotherapy

C. exploratory laparotomy

2. E. omentectomy

4. B. cholecystectomy

Pathology

REVIEW: PATHOLOGY LANGUAGE

I. MATCHING.
F. jaundice
B. curettage
D. gangrene
E. putrefaction
G. cholesterol

2. J. necrosis
4. I. biopsy
6. C. FNA
8. A. cachexia
10. H. washing

II. MULTIPLE CHOICE.
skin
eye/special senses
male reproductive

2. skeletal
4. skin

III. TRUE/FALSE.
false
false
false

2. true
4. false

IV. SPELLING.
Clostridium difficile OR difficile
electrolyte
microscopy
atelectasis
hypernephroma

2. differential
4. reproducibility
6. berylliosis
8. ossification
10. erythrocyte sedimentation OR sedimentation

PATHOLOGY REPORTS 1–3

I. SPELLING.
muscularis
superficial
infiltrate

2. duodenal
4. inflammation

II. MULTIPLE CHOICE.
Helicobacter
villous
serosa

2. mucosa
4. formalin

PATHOLOGY REPORTS 4–5

I. SPELLING.
malignant
aggregating
intracellular

2. carcinoma
4. keratin

II. MATCHING.
C. polyp
B. necrosis
A. pleomorphic

2. E. mitotic
4. D. squamous

PATHOLOGY REPORT 6

I. SPELLING.

epithelial

dilated

edema

2. pathological

4. margins

II. FILL IN THE BLANK.

dysplastic

exocervical

epithelium

2. cone

4. secretory

PATHOLOGY REPORTS 7–9

I. SPELLING.

sweat glands OR sweat

inclusion

hidradenitis

2. fibrosis

4. suppurative

II. MULTIPLE CHOICE.

spermatocele

adenomatous

keratin

2. pseudostratified

4. ellipse

PATHOLOGY REPORTS 10–11

I. SPELLING.

conception

placenta

histology

2. vessels

4. chorionic villi OR chorionic

II. MATCHING.

D. erythropoiesis

A. syncytial

B. hemorrhage

2. E. cotyledon

4. C. necrosis

PATHOLOGY REPORTS 12–13

I. SPELLING.

dermal

entirety

fibroadipose

2. neoplasm

4. specimen

II. MULTIPLE CHOICE.

aggregate

infiltrating

hyperchromatic

2. desmoplasia

4. localization

PATHOLOGY REPORTS 14–16

I. SPELLING.

cartilage

embedded

formalin

2. fragment

4. lateral

II. MATCHING.

B. postauricular

D. collagen

C. follicle

2. E. parakeratosis

4. A. scar

PATHOLOGY REPORT 17

I. SPELLING.

caseating

resuscitation

histologically

2. postmortem

4. adrenals

II. MULTIPLE CHOICE.

subarachnoid

autolysis

capillaries

2. cirrhosis

4. nucleus